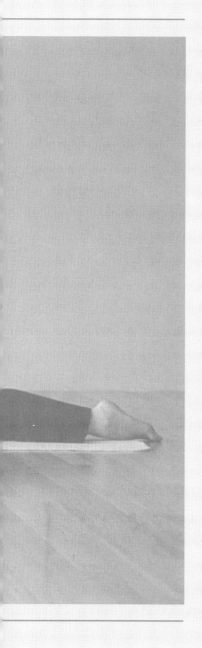

PeeWee Pilates®

Essential
Postpartum
Exercise for
Mother and
Baby

Holly Jean Cosner
and Stacy Malin, Ph.D.

Copyright 2006 © by Holly Jean Cosner and Stacy Malin
Photographs 2006 © Jonathan Pozniak

Designed by Brent Wilcox
Set in 11.5 point New Baskerville by The Perseus Books Group

Library of Congress Cataloging-in-Publication Data
Cosner, Holly Jean.
    PeeWee pilates : essential postpartum exercise for mother and baby / Holly Jean Cosner and Stacy Malin.—1st Da Capo Press ed.
        p.   cm.
    ISBN-13: 978-0-7382-1029-2 (pbk. original : alk. paper)
    ISBN-10: 0-7382-1029-3 (pbk. original : alk. paper) 1. Pilates method. 2. Exercise for women. 3. Exercise for children. 4. Mothers—Health and hygiene. 5. Infants—Care. I. Malin, Stacy. II. Title.
    RA781.4.C67 2005
    613.7'1082—dc22

                                                                        2005022390

First Da Capo Press edition 2006

Published by Da Capo Press
A Member of the Perseus Books Group
http://www.dacapopress.com

Da Capo Press books are available at special discounts for bulk purchases in the U.S. by corporations, institutions, and other organizations. For more information, please contact the Special Markets Department at the Perseus Books Group, 11 Cambridge Center, Cambridge, MA 02142, or call (800) 255-1514 or (617) 252-5298, or email special.markets@perseusbooks.com.

1 2 3 4 5 6 7 8 9—09 08 07 06

PeeWee Pilates®

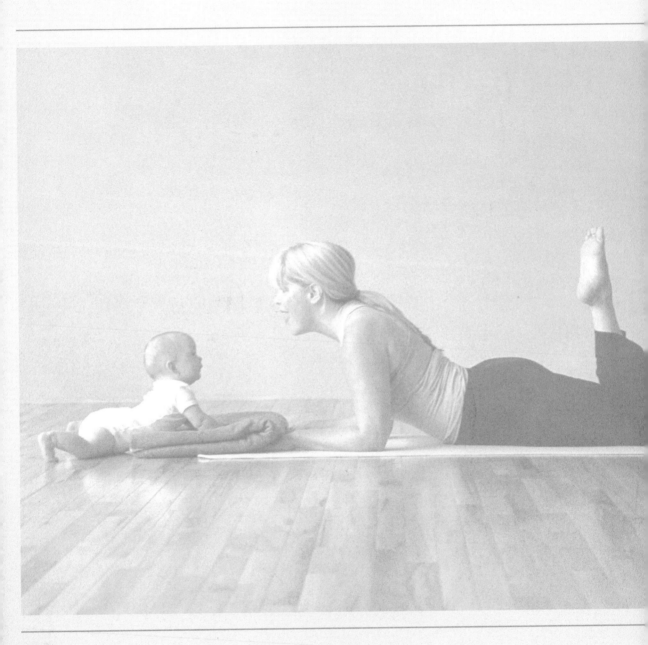

Da Capo
∞
LIFE
LONG

DA CAPO LIFELONG BOOKS
A Member of the Perseus Books Group

HJC: To Tyme, Kai, and Charly,
and to my dad, Michael Cosner, the captain of my world. Love, Holly.

SM: To my own two precious PeeWees, Zoe and Jonas.

Contents

Introduction

First let us offer our congratulations! Your body has just pulled off its most spectacular feat, the creation and delivery of your baby. Those wearing months of pregnancy, the stress of labor and delivery, and those dizzying first few days at home with your newborn are finally behind you. Ahead of you now is the fun part: getting to bond with your sweet little son or daughter!

Now for the less fortunate news: Your body failed to get the memo that it's supposed to snap right back to its prepregnancy state. Instead, your belly has probably become mushy and weak, you may have aches in your back or hips that you never felt before, and your posture is slouchy from all that extra weight you've been carrying around. And let's not forget chronic exhaustion, which seems to have become a permanent new bedfellow.

Welcome to motherhood! Now what?

Some of you disheartened moms vow that the first free moment you get, you're going to throw yourself into a rigorous, five-hour-a-day, boot-camp-style workout to get your old body back. The only problem is that you are still waiting for your free moment to show up.

For some of you new moms, your frumpy state of affairs is nothing new. You weren't exactly a swimsuit model before you became pregnant and you feel even more out of shape now. The prospect of working out has become more intimidating than ever; what was back then a hill to climb is now a steep mountain. What else can you do but subscribe to the mantra: *Should you get the urge to work out, lie down until it passes!* ("I wonder how many calories I can burn changing a diaper?")

Some mothers rationalize that their own beleaguered body is the necessary price of motherhood. Whereas your own body may feel tired, stretched out, and yearning for days gone by, your baby's body radiates with its aura of miracle and hope and endless possibility. Her perfect little toes, delicious smell, and utter enchantment with you are too captivating right now for you to worry about your own figure. Besides, how many times have you heard that your interactions with your baby during those first few months of life will profoundly affect her emotional and physical well-being years later? How can you miss out on that just for tighter abs?

Regardless of your current expectations for your body and your previous fitness level, the reality is that getting moving again after giving birth is rarely easy. The gym might as well be across the ocean, since for some new mothers it feels completely inaccessible. You may only have a babysitter for a few hours or no child care at all, it may be too hard to get there with your baby in tow, or you may not feel like moving, *period*. Night after night of interrupted sleep may leave you more likely to dream about a plush hotel bed than a full-service gym. Running your own twenty-four-hour diner is depleting. Recovering from a C-section or a complicated episiotomy requires patience. And if you were one of those unlucky moms who had to go on bed rest or avoid all exertion at some point in your pregnancy, you may now have an especially long way to go to rebuild stamina.

Getting moving is no guarantee that your body, especially your midsection, will significantly change. Although almost any form of fitness, from spinning to kickboxing, can help you regain endurance and strength, your belly may nonetheless fail to bounce back as obediently as you'd expected. The other problem is that not every exercise is appropriate for postpartum women. For example, your joints remain fragile for months after giving birth, and workouts could end up causing more damage than good if they are too jarring.

This is where PeeWee Pilates comes in.

With PeeWee Pilates, you can begin to significantly renovate your body, especially your pregnancy-battered midsection, practically within weeks of giving birth, without leaving your baby behind. As you tone, tighten, and realign your body, PeeWee Pilates invites your baby to come along for the ride. Literally! You get to incorporate your little son or daughter into the exercises themselves, rolling, lifting, and seesawing together, and, at the same time, tame your torso. What a great opportunity to play with and stimulate your baby while she simultaneously adds challenge and stimulation to your workout! Don't let the fact that your baby is an active participant, however, fool you into thinking that PeeWee Pilates is not a serious, focused workout. In short, concentrated, highly efficient bursts of time, PeeWee Pilates can make a huge difference in how you look, feel, and carry yourself.

PeeWee Pilates is based on the classic Pilates Method and also borrows from yoga techniques, modified so that all the movements target your postpartum needs. We stay true to the Pilates Method by focusing on strengthening your "powerhouse," that is, your abdomen, hips, lower back, and buttocks, the areas that are most strained by pregnancy and new motherhood. Pilates can restore your flexibility, alignment, and balance, all of which are likely to have taken a beating from your pregnancy. You also gain strength in your "core" to help you resist and counter injury and strain from lifting and carrying your baby. The exercises are all designed to be especially kind to your worn joints. The stretching and deep breathing that are a part of each exercise also help combat the day-to-day stresses that accompany parenthood.

The beauty of PeeWee Pilates is that you can do it in the privacy of your home at any time that works well for you and your baby. You don't have to worry about packing up your baby's paraphernalia, donning some flattering workout clothes that camouflage your body, and rushing madly to get to a class at some arbitrary hour that happens to coincide with your baby's nap time. All you need is a mat, two blankets, a small window of opportunity, and your baby. If your baby is a willing, cooperative partner for even just ten- or fifteen-minute bursts of time, your PeeWee Pilates movements can yield results. Some playful tricks to help keep your baby engaged during your workout are offered in Chapter 6 and throughout the exercises.

PeeWee Pilates is a program that can offer significant benefit to almost every postpartum woman. It doesn't matter if you have been a Pilates enthusiast for many years and even kept it up every day of your pregnancy or if you are the quintessential couch potato who thought until now that Pilates was a man in the Bible. You get to decide just how much you feel ready to exert yourself, taking into account your baby's age and ability and your own energy level, experience, and motivation. The mother-baby exercises in the book are relevant at least until your baby is actively and insistently mobile, and for some pairs, beyond your baby's first birthday.

PeeWee Pilates grew out of a collaboration between Holly Jean Cosner, a former professional dancer and a certified instructor in Pilates and Baby Om (a mother-and-baby yoga practice), and one of her clients, Dr. Stacy Malin. Trained by both Romana Kryzanowska, a protégé of Joseph Pilates, and Bob Liekens, a highly regarded master teacher-trainer, Holly has been teaching Pilates in New York City for almost ten years. More recently, she received certification in the Baby Om technique of mother-and-baby yoga from its creators, Laura Staton and Sarah Perron. Stacy Malin is a clinical psychologist and psychoanalyst in full-time private practice in New York City who has worked with parenting issues, body image struggles, and eating disorders for almost two decades. To ensure the safety of both mother and baby, we also consulted with two board-certified physicians, an obstetrician-gynecologist, Dr. Shereen Russell, and a pediatrician, Dr. Natalie Geary, both of whom are in private practice in New York City. Using all our collective expertise, we have created a workout program that aims to do a lot more than just transform your physique. PeeWee Pilates is designed to help you feel more in control and accepting of your own postpartum body. We want you to remember the amazing stunt that your body just pulled off—housing, nurturing, developing, and giving birth to a baby—so that you can appreciate and be kind to your body. We want you to successfully resist joining the 56[1] to 80 percent majority[2] of all the women in this country who are plagued by feelings of dissatisfaction with their appearance. What's at stake here is not just about you. It is important now to take good emotional and physical care of your own body in order to become a more nurturing, supportive caretaker and role model for your baby. Babies who experience their mothers as attuned, happy in their presence, reliable, and comfortable with themselves are more likely to develop a healthy attachment to their mother and enhanced self-esteem.[3]

You have another huge reason to feel good about yourself when you perform PeeWee Pilates. While you are busy executing your Pilates movements with your baby as your partner, you are also actively nurturing your infant's emotional, cognitive, and physical development. Infant research has shown that when babies are massaged, rocked, jiggled, and bounced within the context of a warm interpersonal connection with their mother, they can make great leaps in the development of their motor skills, visual alertness, memory, and sensory discrimination, to name just a few gains. In Chapter 3 and throughout the exercises, you will learn how your baby's development is being enriched as he joins along.

As you turn now to PeeWee Pilates, congratulate yourself on strengthening not only your abdominal core but also your core relationship with your baby. Give yourself a hand for embarking on the ultimate balancing act: meeting the challenge of taking care of your baby while also taking care of *you*!

Part I

You and Your
New Baby

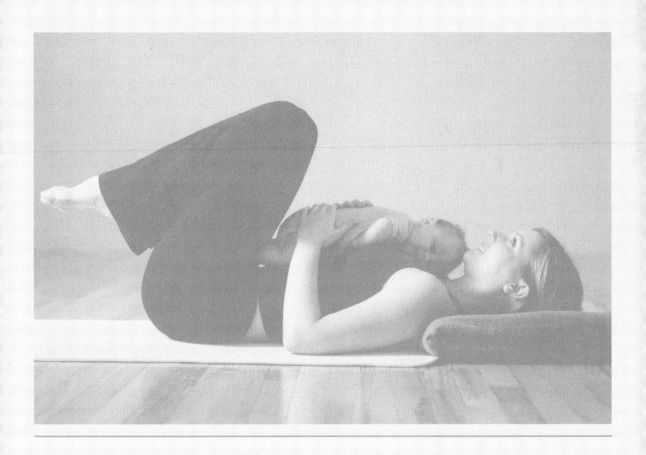

chapter 1

Potbelly and All
Targeting the Physical Needs
of the New Mom

*"Giving birth is like taking your lower lip and
forcing it over your head."*

———————————

Carol Burnett

With the hardship of pregnancy and childbirth now a far distant
memory (sort of) and the haze and havoc of those first few days
home from the hospital starting to clear, it's time to take a fresh look at
yourself. Unfortunately, what you see and feel may not be so pretty. While
many weeks or even months have passed since you gave birth and your
child is already starting to smile, hold his neck up, or even roll over, your
own body may feel as if it is stuck in a postpartum standstill. Forget about
the fantasy that all it would take was a few weeks home from the hospital
for your old jeans to glide over your newly flattened tummy. Wake up and
smell the diaper rash cream! Your stomach still sags down past your hips,
and your buttocks feel as wide as a sumo wrestler's. Your joints feel wobbly.

Your balance is a little off. Loosened ligaments, flabby thighs, and previously unknown aches and pains, not to mention unwanted pounds, may have set up camp in your body like annoying houseguests that just won't take a hint and split. Even with all the awe, excitement, and focus on your new baby, your entire state of mind can be dragged down by the less than fabulous state of your body.

Stretch Marks Are the Least of It: The Wear and Tear of Pregnancy, Childbirth, and Early Parenthood on the New Mom

But wait a minute. Remember the ordeal your body just endured? During the forty weeks that you carried your baby from conception through birth, every aspect of your body went through major upheaval, literally from your head right down to your toes. In case you have already developed a full-blown case of pregnancy amnesia, let's just quickly go through the rundown:

While you were pregnant:

- your **blood volume** increased by about 2¾ pounds, or at least 20 percent
- your **circulatory system** set up hundreds of new capillaries to accommodate the increased blood flow in your body
- your **blood pressure** dropped
- your **blood cholesterol level** increased by about 25–40 percent
- your **hormone levels** surged, with your **estrogen level** alone increasing twenty to forty times
- your **skin** may have developed strange colorations on your face and body, and your **hair** may have changed in both texture and volume

- Your body produced high levels of hormones, particularly relaxin, that softened the connective tissue throughout your body, from your bowels to your lungs, in preparation for childbirth
- your **ligaments**, especially in the hips, abdomen, and pelvis, became overstretched to accommodate your growing baby, and this stretching, in turn, caused the **joints**, which are supported by the ligaments, to become loose or unstable
- your **body weight** increased (most likely) by at least twenty to forty pounds, with at least a pound coming from breast tissue alone
- your **uterus** expanded to a thousand times its normal size
- your **center of gravity** was thrown off kilter because of your increased breast size and your big belly, so your natural alignment was thrown out of whack
- under the pressure of all that extra weight, your **feet** may have expanded by as much as a full shoe size, your **back** may have been strained, and your **posture** likely became more hunched and rounded

And then came baby. Now that it's behind you, let's call a spade a spade. Labor and delivery are no easy feat. The "ship-in-a-bottle" magic trick of pushing your seven-pound, twenty-inch-long baby (on average) out through the usually minuscule opening of your cervix and vaginal canal was not accomplished by smoke and mirrors. A great deal of hard work and pain was required. Your cervix alone needed to dilate to the size of a bagel (about three and a half to four inches across).[1] Add to that the brutal beating that your perineum (the space between your vagina and your anus) had to withstand from your labor. Regardless of whether you wound up having an episiotomy or sustained perineal tearing, your pelvis underwent considerable stress. If you had a cesarean section, you had to contend with a whole different kind of ordeal, namely, major abdominal surgery with incisions in both your abdomen and your uterus. Your guts were pulled apart, and your uterus was literally removed from your body and had to be put back in its proper place.

And guess what? Surprise, surprise! The physical demands of mother-hood do not end with childbirth. On the contrary, as we're sure you've al-ready discovered, mothering a young infant can be shockingly physically taxing. Just when your weakened body is in the process of recovering, you are being called upon 24/7 to diaper, nurse, pace, soothe, lift, bend, wash, wipe, rock, cradle, and tolerate bloodcurdling cries. These innocent mater-nal tasks carry all sorts of occupational hazards, from low back strain to neck pain to tennis elbow to pure exhaustion. If you're nursing your baby, please add to the list cracked nipples, cramped and rounded shoulders, and upper back pain, among other ailments.

Exercise: The Prescription for Postpartum Recovery

With the intense toll that pregnancy, childbirth, and new motherhood have taken on both your body and your mental state, the simple passage of time is not going to do the trick to put it all back on track. Your body is going to need some help. What kind? You guessed it: good old-fashioned exercise. Exercise does not just get your heart pumping. For new moms, exercise can accelerate physical recovery and the maintenance of overall health. Post-partum exercise has been linked to improvements in aerobic fitness (i.e., the ability to use oxygen more efficiently), HDL cholesterol levels (your good cholesterol), and insulin sensitivity.[2]

Ironically, it is in the first year after giving birth that women have a par-ticularly difficult time pursuing a regular exercise program. In one study, 40 percent of new moms who were enrolled in a year-long structured exercise program for postpartum women dropped out well before the study was completed.[3] Apparently, even highly motivated women were unable to commit because of competing parenting and work demands. We don't have to tell you that caring for an infant is an incredibly time-consuming and lifestyle-altering affair.

PeeWee Pilates: The All-Around Powerhouse Postpartum Solution

In order for a postpartum exercise program to be effective, it must be mindful of the new mother's unique laundry list of vulnerabilities, risks, and needs. Pregnancy and its aftermath are a whole-body experience worthy of a holistic approach to recovery. A new mom needs a highly flexible exercise regimen that attends to the "whole person" (as opposed to just specific body parts), that is tolerant of her changing physical limitations and needs, that takes into account her considerable time constraints, that can adjust for the ever-present fatigue of motherhood, that incorporates some relaxation techniques, and that promotes an overall improved sense of psychological and physical well-being.

That is where PeeWee Pilates comes in. PeeWee Pilates is the first Pilates exercise program created to specifically target the bodies of postpartum women. We emphasize a flexible, easily modifiable approach to fitness that matches your exercises to the vulnerabilities and strengths of your progressively recovering postpartum body and your shifting state of mind. Exercises are varied in terms of level of difficulty, intensity, concentration, and length of time. This way, you tackle only as much as you feel prepared to handle at any particular point depending upon fluctuations in your energy, mood, time allowance, and physical strength. All of the movements can be performed right in your own bedroom or living room, so you don't have to worry about making it to a gym. And if you need yet another reason to work out at home, consider this: Several studies have confirmed that people who exercise *at home* are more likely to maintain their workout over time and lose more weight to boot.[4]

Although cardiovascular activities like running and weight training can be fantastic workouts for rebuilding strength and endurance, overdoing it can cause unnecessary injury. Bouncing or jarring movements can easily result in strains, sprains, and other damage to your weakened joints. When resuming postpartum exercise, it is important not to overstress these loose joints and stretched-out ligaments, which can remain unstable for a few months postchildbirth. Relaxin, the hormone secreted during pregnancy, continues to affect your body for at least three months postnatally,[5] so your muscles, joints, and ligaments may all remain softened during this time. A goal of Pilates is to strengthen and tighten the muscular area around your overstressed joints or ligaments, rather than to work directly on and further tax these body parts. By moving your body gently and precisely within its natural alignment, you will prevent your joints from locking or straining and simultaneously encourage the muscles to work more deliberately to support the joints.

But let's face it. What most new mothers want from an exercise program has nothing to do with joints and ligaments. What most new mothers want is to look attractive and sexy again, and PeeWee Pilates is on the case! PeeWee Pilates gets to work right away to restore your almighty "powerhouse" midsection or core, the part of your body most strained by pregnancy. *The powerhouse is the group of muscles surrounding the body from the mid thigh up to the tips of the shoulder blades.* This section includes the muscles around your hips, inner thighs, pelvic floor, and rib cage as well as all the back muscles. And, of course, let us not exclude the abdominal muscles, those powerful, elastic bands of crisscrossing muscle fiber that make up the bulk of the powerhouse. Strengthening and tightening this group of muscles will go a long way toward flattening and toning your middle. At the same time, it will enhance support for your back and improve your alignment, balance, and flexibility.

Postpartum Trouble Spots

Let's look more closely at how PeeWee Pilates will zero in on those annoying postpregnancy problems.

The Shock of the Jelly Belly: Abdominal Muscles

Your abdominal muscles, which represent the most significant aspect of the powerhouse, bore the biggest brunt of your pregnancy wear and tear. Your uterus lies just beneath your abdominal wall; as it expanded over the course of your pregnancy, sheltering your growing baby and the placenta, your abdominal muscles and ligaments both obviously had to stretch considerably to accommodate all that growth. It takes about six weeks after giving birth for your uterus to shrink naturally back to its prepregnancy size. (Breastfeeding can help speed up the process.) Unfortunately, your abdominal muscles don't bounce back quite so readily. Three different muscle groups—the rectus abdominis, the obliques, and the transverse muscles—comprise your abdominal muscles; none of these escaped the wrath of your big nine-month-old belly. Your rectus abdominis are the muscles that, in an ideal world, give you that six-pack look and lift your upper body. The internal and external obliques are those muscles that help you twist and bend. During your pregnancy, these skeletal muscles were stretched and pushed out and to the side. Doing crunches will offer some help to strengthen these muscles but will not significantly engage your transverse muscles. The transverse muscles are that deepest layer of muscle that completely wraps around your body, enabling your torso to potentially rotate in a 360-degree circle. These are the muscles that you can sometimes feel when you cough, laugh, or exhale deeply, and they are perhaps the most important for providing core abdominal strength and for cinching in your entire waist. PeeWee Pilates simultaneously corrects all three muscle groups in almost every one of its powerhouse-strengthening exercises. Unfortunately, your overstretched abdominal ligaments do not possess much elasticity and will not respond as readily to exercise. However, as your abdominal muscles tighten, they will pull your overstretched abdominal ligaments tighter around you, giving you a smoother, flatter tummy.

We should mention that there are many other reasons besides flattening your stomach that should motivate you to strive for stronger abdominal muscles. Abdominal strength can markedly alleviate and prevent backaches and at the same time dramatically improve your balance. The key to balance, in fact, is a strong powerhouse. It can also reduce the risk of developing varicose veins, leg cramps, edema, and formation of blood clots in the veins. Strong abdominal muscles have even been credited with helping to maintain urinary continence, since they help support part of the pelvis in the front of your body.[6]

The Case of the Bottom Falling Out: Pelvic Floor

If you had a vaginal delivery, your pelvic floor is experiencing a temporary case of post-traumatic stress disorder! As Dr. Russell, our consulting ob-gyn, described it, the pelvic floor is a "trampoline of muscles" that holds together the vaginal wall, the rectum, and the urethra. With a vaginal birth, all three layers of muscles are traumatized. The muscles around your vagina get stretched, and your bladder can start to fall in. Do not underestimate the power and punch of your pelvic muscles! They work as a team to keep your abdominal and pelvic organs properly supported and positioned, they help you maintain continence (i.e., so you don't urinate unintentionally), and last but not least, they may even enhance sexual pleasure for both you and your partner. That's enough reason to take it seriously! During the course of your pregnancy, your pelvic floor had the unenviable job of helping to hold your uterus in place, baby, big belly, and all. Between the strain of this task, the softening of the pelvic floor muscles from the elevated hormones, and the trauma to the pelvic floor from the vaginal delivery, after you've given birth your pelvic muscles have become devastatingly weakened. This weakness does not even include the potential damage to your pelvic area from the commonly performed episiotomy.

If you are experiencing any urinary leakage, the culprit is most likely weakened pelvic floor muscles. Urinary incontinence is a common nuisance during pregnancy, especially during the last trimester, but can continue for months after childbirth. Many new mothers are quite dismayed to encounter ongoing problems with mild to moderate urinary incontinence when they exert themselves in the slightest way. Squatting, sneezing, or even laughing can be enough for you to lose control of your urine. If you were feeling particularly antsy to start running or kickboxing or engaging in some other high-intensity workout, urinary incontinence can become quite a deterrent. One study found that 30 percent of women who exercised regularly complained of urinary leakage; 20 percent of these women were bothered enough to abandon their workouts.[7]

All of the PeeWee Pilates exercises that engage the lower part of the powerhouse will be working to strengthen and tighten your pelvic floor muscles. Kegel exercises, in which you engage and squeeze the pelvic muscles, are also a must. In fact, because Kegels are so essential to strengthening your pelvic floor, we want to encourage you to consider them your daily warm-up for Pilates. Make sure that you review in Chapter 7 exactly how to perform Kegels correctly.

The Not-So-Sweet Swayback: Alignment and Posture

Even the woman with the most superb posture and form experiences a profound shift in balance and alignment during the course of her pregnancy and can benefit enormously from corrective work postpartum. Remember that as your baby grew inside you, your entire center of gravity shifted. Picture an imaginary line extending from the top of your head straight down to your feet. Before you got pregnant, and assuming you possessed good natural alignment, your ears lined up directly over your shoulders and your hips balanced over the arches of your feet. Over the course of your pregnancy, however, as your belly and breasts grew exponentially, this line completely shifted, and your hips were now balanced over the front of your toes. At the same time, your hips, pelvis, and buttocks softened and widened to accommodate your increased weight and to prepare for childbirth. To compensate for all these changes, your body had to make many other adjustments. Your feet spread farther apart and turned out slightly to offset your shift in balance, giving your gait the appearance of a duck waddle. Under the pressure of this increased weight, your shoulders also tended to round forward and your lower back may have tended to arch, creating a condition called swayback, or lumbar lordosis. Low back pain is a complaint among at least 50 percent of all pregnant women. (It didn't help that you had no opportunity during the latter part of your pregnancy to stretch out your lower back with either forward bends or counterstretches, because of the positioning of your baby in utero.) Your weight gain also placed a strain on your hips, knees, ankles, and feet that further distorted your entire natural alignment. Your alignment does not automatically reverse to its prepregnant state after childbirth. It has to be worked on.

Unfortunately, good posture and alignment remain in constant jeopardy as you go about the hectic business of caring for a young infant. Bending over a crib to scoop up your baby and nursing your infant in a hunched-over position are two instances where damage to your back, neck, and shoulders can impair your alignment. One of the most common threats to good alignment comes from trying to juggle your baby on one arm while freeing your other to handle the five million other things you need to be doing at the same time. If you are like most moms, you tend to carry your baby around on your left arm with the baby resting against your hip. Your right hand is thus freed to grab the phone, brush your hair, put the dishes in the sink, pick up toys, and maybe even hold your other child's hand. To add insult to injury, you may even have the extra weight of your diaper bag dangling over that same shoulder. Sound familiar? Unfortunately, this asymmetry leaves you at risk for throwing your hips out of alignment, overdeveloping and shortening the muscles on the right side of your body, straining your joints, and putting pressure on your probably overarched lower back. This repeated misalignment, in turn, could wreak havoc on your neck and right shoulder and trigger pain in your back that could migrate down to your hip, knee, ankle, and even your foot. If you favor one side habitually, you may be well on your way to developing a scoliosis of the spine or an unattractive, crooked stride that leaves you vulnerable to even more injury!

PeeWee Pilates focuses intensively on correcting your alignment. Each exercise trains your body to move within the natural limits of your own skeletal frame. Your muscles are encouraged to work evenly and uniformly to reinforce good form. As you practice Pilates, you will become increasingly aware of your own alignment and recognize when you are not in conformity with it. By shifting your hips and shoulders back into alignment, you can undo limb, back, and joint strain and reduce your risk of additional injury.

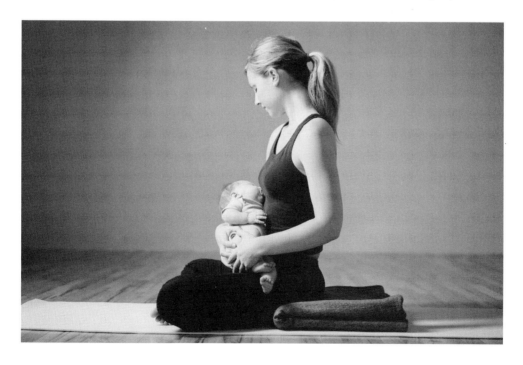

The F Word: How Pilates Can Help You Begin to
Take Control of Your Weight

Right now you're probably feeling a bit on the flabby side. How could you not? It's impossible for any woman, even one who works out fanatically right through her pregnancy, to avoid losing at least some muscle tone over the course of those nine months. Even more disconcerting for new mothers is that layer of fat covering their postpartum body that just didn't reside there a year before. That layer is actually to be expected. While you were pregnant, your body was squirreling away body fat, both to support your baby's needs during pregnancy and to build your milk supply for your baby. Thanks to elevations in progesterone throughout your pregnancy, a lot of this fat got stored in the lower part of your body, especially from the waist down.[8] Just how much fat is stored away varies from woman to woman. Some of you may have been so scrupulous about your diet during your pregnancy that you barely gained enough weight to keep your obstetrician happy. On the other hand, some of you may have treated pregnancy as an opportunity to loosen up your belt and at long last indulge! On the bright side, you should remember that the average new mother returns relatively quickly to within a few pounds of her prepregnancy weight, especially if she just gave birth to her first child. The majority of women lose between seventeen and twenty pounds soon after the birth,[9] and shed almost all their pregnancy weight within the first three months after delivery. Unfortunately, however, not every woman is so lucky. As unfair as it may seem, some new mothers, especially those who gained a lot of extra weight during their pregnancy, tend to experience childbirth as a prelude to a lifetime of extra pounds and even obesity. Giving birth to a baby increases your risk of becoming moderately overweight by 60 percent and becoming obese by 110 percent![10] In her book *Pregnancy Weight Management* (2000), Francis-Cheung offers many reasons for postpartum weight gain. They include the difficulty of readjusting your food intake for one rather than two, concerns about getting enough nutrients for breast-feeding, eating to feed your stressful feelings, and the metabolic changes that accompany childbirth. She also notes that the higher ratio of fat tissue to muscle mass in the early postpartum period slows down your metabolic rate, leading to either weight gain or a slowdown in weight loss. If you are breast-feeding, your metabolic rate may also slow down to ensure adequate fat storage for your milk supply. Many women fall prey to the misconception that if they are breast-feeding, they will lose all their pregnancy weight spontaneously. Unfortunately, this just isn't so. Breast-feeding has little impact on postpartum weight loss, presumably because nursing mothers tend to compensate by increasing their caloric intake and decreasing their activity level.[11]

So How Can Pilates Help? Being physically active after giving birth (especially in conjunction with a sensible nutritional program!) may promote weight loss.[12] Although aerobic exercises like running or cycling are a great way to burn fat, they are not always feasible for new mothers, and they are certainly not sufficient to meet the bodily needs of the postpartum woman. Weak joints, low energy, lack of muscle strength, urinary incontinence (as noted earlier), and lack of a babysitter can all get in the way of a vigorous mid-morning jog. As a weight-bearing activity, Pilates is a great way to regain strength and stamina. You get to build muscle while you protect your joints. Because muscles use up more energy than fat, as you gain muscle, you will increase your metabolism and encourage weight loss. Pilates guides you to strengthen and elongate your muscles using the natural resistance created by the weight of your own body as you lift and pull against it. With PeeWee Pilates, you add even more weight—the extra pounds of your baby! Lifting and moving with your baby definitely intensifies your strength training. Strengthening and elongating your muscles is the key to toning and redefining your body. Throughout the Pilates exercises, you will be instructed to move your body as if you're underwater. Moving with this slow intention and against your own resistance tightens the muscle to the bone and creates tone. With Pilates, movements always entail deliberate, focused squeezing and engaging of the muscles while making sure not to hyperextend or lock the joints. And don't forget that the powerhouse is fortified with each and every Pilates exercise. What this means is that the muscles in your abdomen, back, butt, hips, and thighs are all getting a workout with each Pilates movement.

Gasping for Air: Breathing

Taking in a big breath should be something you take for granted. During the latter part of your pregnancy, however, as your uterus enlarged and pushed up on the diaphragm, it crowded the lungs and made it difficult for your lungs to expand fully. In addition, because of the pregnancy hormones, the capillaries of the respiratory tract swelled up and the muscles of the lungs and bronchial tubes relaxed. The result of all this is that your breathing became much more shallow during your pregnancy. Your lungs had to work overtime to breathe in 40–50 percent more air to increase your oxygen supply for your unborn baby, and yet your own brain received a significant drop in oxygen (perhaps contributing to that lightheadedness you might have experienced).

One of the first things you can do after having your baby is start working on your "Pre-Hundreds Breathing" (see page 86). Breathing properly is an essential aspect of any Pilates workout. With proper breathing, you can improve your stamina, relax both your mind and your muscles, increase your lung capacity, enhance your circulation, and energize your whole body. That is not all. The deep breathing that accompanies the movements can actually help you to detoxify your body of impurities.

When you inhale deeply, you are oxygenating your entire body, especially your muscles; when you exhale, you are extracting toxins from the body. Inhaling deeply through your nose expands the diaphragm downward and allows more air in; exhaling deeply contracts the diaphragm upward toward the chest and encourages the abdominal muscles to work harder to push out more air. Breathing from their diaphragm is what enables opera singers to hold those long notes. In the same way that deep breathing may have helped you hang in there through those intense hours (or minutes for those lucky few) in labor and delivery, the Pilates breath will help carry you through your postpartum Pilates workout. For those of you who are familiar with yoga, meditation, weight training, running, or other forms of fitness and relaxation techniques, the importance of the breath is nothing new.

A Tale of Two Ta-Tas: Your Ever-Changing Breasts

Almost no body part undergoes as much transformation during pregnancy, childbirth, and the postpartum period as your breasts! Practically from the moment you became pregnant, one of the very first signs you may have noticed that something was cooking inside you was your swollen, tender breasts. Much to some mothers' delight and other women's horror, over the course of a pregnancy, the breasts continue to expand, as fatty tissue, glandular tissue, and an elaborate milk-producing network, including alveoli and milk ducts, sets up shop inside. Even more unexpected for many of you are the profound changes that your breasts undergo right after childbirth. You certainly don't need to be reminded about those early postpartum days; your breasts were painfully engorged, you leaked milk all over your favorite shirt, or your bra size increased by two, three, or even more sizes. Regardless of whether you chose to breast-feed, your breasts await more changes in the postpartum period. Most women experience a loss in firmness, a drop in perkiness, and a change in breast size (either larger or smaller than usual) for several months after childbirth or after breast-feeding. (Interestingly, breast-feeding has not been found to be responsible for breast sagginess; the real culprit is genetics, the toll of pregnancy itself, and its accompanying weight gain.)[13] Although your breasts may never fully return to their prepregnancy size or shape, the good news is that within about a year, the skin around your breasts is likely to firm up again.[14]

So how can Pilates help?

- Pilates is a great form of exercise for breast-feeding moms. Its focus on posture and alignment can encourage women to assume a more comfortable nursing position. One common reason why mothers can get sore nipples is incorrect positioning. Pilates encourages nursing mothers to open up their chests by strengthening their shoulder muscles and pectorals. Kyphosis, or a forward rounding of the back, is a common problem for nursing mothers, which Pilates will go to work to correct.

- The emphasis in Pilates on strengthening muscles may be helpful in preventing or slowing down the loss in bone density that can accompany breast-feeding. Nursing moms commonly suffer from a temporary loss of bone-mineral density. Studies have consistently found changes in axial bone loss ranging from 3 percent to 9 percent over periods of time as short as two to six months.[15]

- Some extremely high-intensity forms of exercise may alter the content of breast milk and make it taste less desirable to babies. What happens is that lactic acid can build in the body from intense exercise and, in turn, can elevate the acidity in the milk.[16] With moderate exercise like Pilates, you don't need to worry about harming the quantity or composition of your breast milk.

Special Delivery: Following a Cesarean Section

One out of every four babies is now delivered by cesarean section, making this the most common surgical procedure performed in the United States.[17] In fact, more and more women are electing to have a scheduled cesarean. Despite the increasing popularity of this surgery, many new mothers who had hoped to have a vaginal delivery experience profound disappointment, regret, and even a sense of failure if they end up having an emergency C-section. Unfortunately, if you had a C-section, you are at greater risk for postpartum depression. At the same time, please be reassured that having a C-section carries its own advantages. For one, your pelvic floor was spared the trauma of a vaginal delivery. Your risk of incontinence, hemorrhoids, and prolapsed organs later in life are all significantly lessened.[18]

There is a great deal of variability in how quickly women recuperate from a cesarean section. Some women are up and out within weeks of delivery, whereas others experience considerable pain and exhaustion over an extended period of time. Many women struggle to lift and hold their baby after a C-section and may have trouble sitting up to breast-feed. Some women even need to lie down while they nurse. Other women complain of numbness around their incision and feel disconnected from their abdominal muscles. After a C-section, some new mothers can't roll up to save their lives.

Because there are so many of you who are recovering from a C-section, we offer a special set of instructions accompanying each exercise that take into account the particular weaknesses and vulnerabilities that can follow a C-section delivery. If you're feeling strong, you can choose to follow the regular instructions. If you are feeling less confident, you may find the C-section modifications plenty challenging.

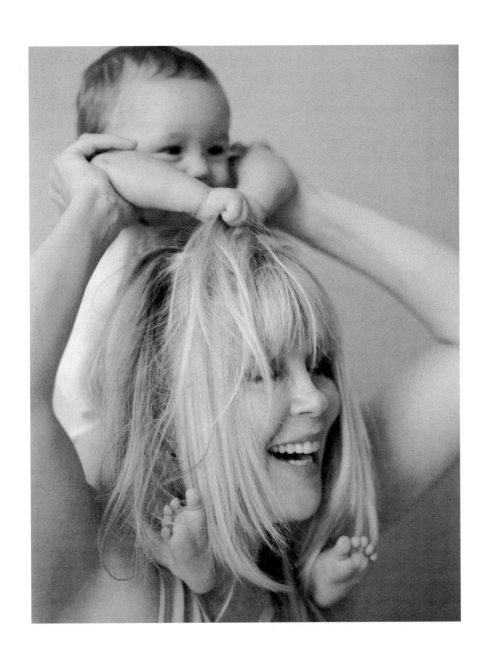

chapter 2

If Mama Ain't Happy
Targeting the Psychological Needs
of the New Mom

"I could see now that having a baby is, pardon the understatement, a crisis—at least until it settles down into being just your life."

Susan Squire, "Maternal Bitch,"
in *The Bitch in the House*, p. 211.

When you have a newborn baby, you don't just introduce an adorable little person into your life; you also bring home with you a swirl of complicated, intense emotions. Regardless of whether you just had your first child or you are on your fourth, your exhilaration and joy over your new family member gets juxtaposed with a whole other set of feelings: loss, disruption, powerlessness, worry, fear, exhaustion, resentment, entrapment, or terror. Just the physical responsibilities of parenting can be surprisingly overwhelming. Although you may have expected that you'd be on call nonstop, you might never have anticipated how hard it would be just to take a shower. For some new mothers, the really hard part

is the transition into the new identity of "mom" and all that this role con-
jures up for each individual woman. Dilemmas such as whether or not to
go back to work or whether or not to breast-feed can degenerate into
huge crises about how you define your very core sense of self. Some
women plague themselves with anxiety or doubt about whether their
mothering skills are living up to their own impossibly high expectations.
Others may be more concerned about their baby's well-being. And how
can you hold this adorable little baby without relating somehow to yourself as a baby? Pleasant early childhood memories may arise alongside
painful ones that you might not have explored before. Bringing a new little player into the family mix also inevitably provokes major changes in
your relationship with your partner. In the months following the birth of
a baby, many couples temporarily "lose" each other; it is all too easy to feel
deserted, unsupported, criticized, or disappointed by your partner's different style of parenting or shifting relationship with you. We haven't even
mentioned yet all those other compounding stresses, such as stretched fi-
nances, the conflicting needs of an older child, a deeply disappointing
birth experience, or health concerns.

At the same time that you're contending with this profound psychological adjustment, you may also be plagued by yet another source of un-
settling feelings, namely, a less than perfect body image. Worries about attractiveness as well as sexual desirability often surface as new mothers
recover from pregnancy. Your swollen breasts, stretch marks, and excess
pounds can all leave you feeling surprisingly inadequate, ashamed, or
damaged and may have an overwhelmingly negative impact on your overall self-esteem.

These psychological challenges are even more difficult to manage when
you are physically not at the top of your game. Your emotional state is already being pummeled by the deadly combination of an abrupt drop in
hormonal level and sleep deprivation.

Blues, Sweat, and Tears:
Postpartum Depression and Other Problems

Not surprisingly, a large majority of new moms are struck with the "baby blues" in the first couple of weeks after childbirth. This is a very brief bout of depression that usually disappears within ten days to two weeks and is characterized by inexplicable crying spells and sudden mood swings. By reminding you, however, just how common the baby blues are, affecting anywhere from 70 to 85 percent of all mothers,[1] and just how quickly they usually resolve, we hope to reassure you not to get too bent out of shape by this short-lived roller-coaster ride.

Unfortunately, however, there is no other time in a woman's life when she is as biologically vulnerable to developing a psychiatric disorder as she is in her first postpartum year. In contrast to the baby blues, a significant percentage of women experience more persistent emotional discomfort. About 10–15 percent of all moms wind up with a more pronounced depression, one that is much more intense and longer lasting.[2] This "postpartum depression" usually surfaces within the first six to eight weeks after giving birth but can actually begin at any point in the first six months to a year following childbirth. A postpartum depression can last for just a few weeks or a few months, but for up to 30–70 percent of all women who suffer, it can hang around for a full year or more. Postpartum depression does not discriminate on the basis of class, age, or education level. In her memoir, *Down Came the Rain* (Hyperion, 2005), well known actress and model Brooke Shields lets us know that even celebrities can be at risk. Shields bravely attempts to tear down the stigma attached to this disorder by candidly sharing her own personal struggle with postpartum depression following the birth of her daughter, Rowan.[3]

How do you recognize a postpartum depression in the making? Symptoms may include:

- Sad mood
- Diminished interest or pleasure in most activities
- Difficulty concentrating
- Feelings of worthlessness or intense guilt
- Tearfulness
- Irritability, impatience, or anger
- Difficulty making decisions
- A fear of being left alone
- Feeling inadequate to take care of your baby
- Insomnia, extreme tiredness, or both
- Wishing that you were dead
- Restlessness
- A sense of emotional numbness
- Less interest in sex
- Excessive concern or lack of concern for your baby
- Withdrawal from family and friends

Many more women experience just a few of the symptoms mentioned above and would not qualify for the diagnosis of a full-blown postpartum depression. Indeed, it is quite common to experience a milder form of depression postpartum.[4] It is also not uncommon to encounter significant anxiety at this point without accompanying depression. Referred to as *postpartum anxiety* or *panic disorder,* this latter condition may show up as strong anxiety and fear, rapid breathing, fast heart rate, hot or cold flashes, chest pain, and shakiness or dizziness.[5] Although these conditions have not received as much attention as postpartum depression, that does not mean that you do not also suffer or are not in need of real help.

When you are depressed, it can be an incredible struggle to get out of bed, let alone provide sensitive and predictable care to your baby. Many mothers can't help but become utterly absorbed by their sadness and may withdraw from or misread the emotional needs of their baby. This does not keep you from worrying about your parenting skills; on the contrary, many women with postpartum depression worry like crazy that they are inadequate as mothers and experience profound guilt.

If you do become depressed after childbirth, the last thing you need to do is to attribute your suffering to some character flaw or weakness within yourself. Unfortunately, one of the symptoms of depression is self-condemnation; you certainly don't need an extra helping of things to feel bad about. Remember, the postpartum deck is stacked with tons of risk factors, many of which can be impossible to sidestep. The physical transformations that occur after childbirth are a major culprit, particularly the abrupt and dramatic drop in estrogen and progesterone and the good possibility of thyroid-related hormonal changes that can make you feel lethargic and depressed. After childbirth, your body is also confronted with alterations affecting your blood volume, blood pressure, immune system, and metabolism. These changes are all quite capable of souring how you feel, emotionally as well as physically. And let's not forget the ramifications of good old-fashioned sleep deprivation; lack of sleep can exacerbate everything, rendering otherwise frustrating but manageable conflicts suddenly completely overwhelming.

Unfortunately, when a mother suffers from an untreated depression, her disorder can also have all sorts of repercussions for her family. When you are depressed, your baby knows it. Your baby is exquisitely attuned to your feelings (see the next chapter); your stress has a powerful effect on your baby. Children who are cared for by a mother with an *untreated* postpartum depression are much more likely to experience disturbances in the mother-infant relationship and are at notably greater risk for the development, even years later, of a wide range of behavioral problems and psychological impairments.[6] These can run the gamut from irregular sleep to delays in verbal abilities and lack of school readiness skills. Please do note that the operative word here is *untreated!* With proper help, the large majority of women who suffer from a postpartum depression respond quite well. Fortunately, a number of different interventions can be extraordinarily effective at combating postpartum depression. Help may include antidepressant medications, hormone therapy (such as an estrogen patch, which counteracts the sudden drop of estrogen following birth), individual insight-oriented psychotherapy, and supportive group therapy.

Lighting the Fire in Your Belly

Regardless of whether you're suffering a postpartum depression or just the stress and turmoil of new parenting, what better way is there to give your psychological health a boost than to take your baby in tow and start moving! Although few doubt that exercise can perk you up, you might be surprised to learn the degree to which postpartum fitness can be a powerful tool to combat emotional distress in new mothers. When new moms work out consistently, they significantly lower their risk of both postpartum depression and anxiety.[7] Postpartum women who exercise also tend to feel less overwhelmed, more prepared to master the challenges of motherhood, and happier with their bodies.[8]

Pilates is an ideal form of exercise to improve one's state of mind. The stretching encourages the release of tensions held in the body, and the coordinated breath discourages unnecessary muscle stress. Deep breathing, we believe, should be a mandatory component of postpartum fitness. Pilates breathing—through the nose—is especially effective at stress reduction. As Dr. Christiane Northrup, a leading obstetrician-gynecologist and recognized advocate for women's health, explains, "When we learn how to breathe fully through our nose, aerating our lower lungs and allowing our rib cage a full expansion, our body relaxes and we experience a sense of peace. . . . I'm convinced that everyone should adopt this method of breathing not only for exercise, but for daily living."[9] Who could benefit more from this breathing than a stressed-out new mom?

Focus and concentration are also a part of every Pilates exercise. As you concentrate on a visual metaphor to help position yourself for each movement, your mind is alert in the present. When stretching, breathing, and focused effort are all performed in synchrony, you are creating a kind of moving meditation.

And let us not forget to mention what can sometimes be the most uplifting aspect of PeeWee Pilates: the opportunity to cuddle and have fun with your baby. The exercises invite you to get down on the floor with your little cutie and engage in direct face-to-face interactions. Seeing your baby's delight in you register on her face as you play together can elicit an unparalleled sense of joy and warmth. Cuddling your baby, too, may be truly intoxicating. It turns out that maintaining body contact (preferably direct skin-to-skin) with your little one may actually produce elevated levels of a peptide hormone called oxytocin in your body that can improve your mood. Discovered by Swedish researchers,[10] oxytocin is believed to promote a feeling of caring, calm, and increased sensitivity in mothers. Referred to as the *bonding hormone*,[11] it has actually been found to lower blood pressure and heart rate. For these reasons, oxytocin has been described as "the endocrinological equivalent of candlelight, soft music and a glass of wine."[12] So cuddle away!

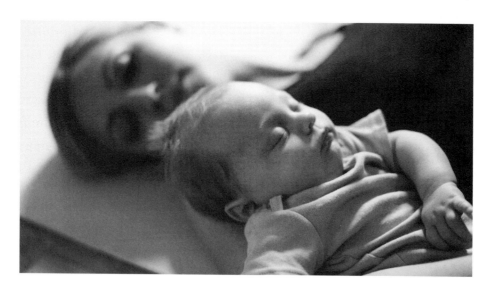

Confessions of a Rundown Goddess: Body Confidence

Will You Ever Feel Attractive Again?

A major source of bad feelings for new moms is the current state of their body. No one has to tell you that feeling badly about how you look is a total downer! Unfortunately, during these postpartum months when you can no longer blame your protruding abs and wide hips on your growing pregnancy, it can be hard to sustain compassion for your own recovering body. Wistfully you wonder if your stretch marks will ever go away (there's actually a new cream that really works!)[13] or if your breasts will ever return to their prepregnancy size and shape or if your hair will stop falling out (a natural temporary reaction to the drop in hormones). Will you ever catch up on enough sleep to reduce the bags under your eyes or perk up that sallow, tired complexion? Will you ever feel attractive again? To watch your little son or daughter blossom from day to day and yet observe little bloom in your own appearance months after giving birth can be extremely frustrating; it is at this significant postpartum juncture that self-criticism and despair unfortunately frequently escalate. One study found that 70 percent of new moms harbored terrible dissatisfaction with their body at six months postpartum, and 39 percent remained dissatisfied one year after childbirth.[14] Sadly, the postpartum period is a time of increased vulnerability for the development of serious body image impairment and eating disorders. (Take note that this risk is especially heightened for women who had been trying to lose weight before they became pregnant.) New mothers who can't seem to drop unwanted pounds or who fear that they're on a crash course toward obesity may become tempted to put themselves on a starvation diet or else throw in the towel and just eat uncontrollably. Either way, women who feel badly about their bodies are at much higher risk for developing a postpartum depression.

Struggling with a poor body image can also affect how we parent. Each and every one of us can't help but communicate nonverbally how we feel in our bodies. Our movements, gestures, posture, and dress speak volumes about how we experience ourselves internally. In turn, our feelings about our bodies can profoundly influence many of our behaviors as a parent. As an example, new moms who harbor a negative body image are much less inclined to breast-feed,[15] perhaps because of their discomfort with or lack of pleasure in their own bodies. Believe it or not, even a small infant can detect subtle unspoken communications by his mother about her own maternal body. For example, babies can sense in some unformed way whether their parents welcome or avoid touch, feel open or stiff, or look engaged or distracted. Part of the danger is that mothers who have trouble embracing their own physical appearance might unintentionally pass their own poor body image on to their children. As young children pick up cues about how their parents regard their own bodies, they may come to attach such beliefs or concerns to their own appearance or sense of self.[16] Unwittingly parents may also impose their own harsh standards about their bodies on their children; for example, the mother who is intolerant of even the slightest personal weight gain may perceive her well-nourished baby as "chubby."

Clearly, regaining your confidence and pleasure in your own body is no trivial matter. It is not just a matter of vanity. Finding value and joy in your *maternal* body is vital. At stake in feeling like a goddess is your total psychological well-being.

Body Image Saboteurs

How would you rate *your* own body confidence during these last few months since giving birth? Take a look at the list below and see how many of the characteristics apply to you since you became a mother. How often do you find that you

- can't help but compare your body to that of every other new mother you see on the street?

- deliberately dress down or cover up your body (e.g., wearing sweats or baggy clothes all the time)?
- avoid social situations because you don't feel good about how you look?
- avoid sex or even just plain physical affection with your partner because you don't feel attractive enough?
- find yourself using your baby as an excuse to overlook fixing your hair or applying makeup?
- interview every mother you know about how long it took her to lose her baby weight and then rebuke yourself if you are taking longer (or, alternatively, feel triumphant if you are "winning")?
- ask others around you incessantly, "Do I look like I'm losing weight?"
- feel compelled to remind every new person that you meet that you just had a baby and "don't usually look like this"?
- scrutinize your waist and butt in the mirror with an evil eye?
- try on your prepregnancy clothes even though you *know* they still don't fit?
- weigh yourself at least once a day but only after you pee?

If any of these behaviors sound a bit too familiar, your body image may have taken a hard hit as you transitioned to motherhood. Fortunately, Pee-Wee Pilates can help revive—or find—the goddess in you. Pilates is an ideal tool to help you regain (or develop for the first time) control of and pleasure in your own body. With regular Pilates practice, it is a common experience to feel one's entire body change in shape. By focusing on elongating the muscles and lengthening the spine, you begin to feel taller and lighter. Your waist especially feels longer and leaner as you start to feel the distance between your hips and shoulders extend. In the strengthening of your powerhouse, your middle also starts to feel increasingly cinched in, as if you are wearing a shape-enhancing corset.

Wouldn't it be cool if we as authors could just snap our fingers and prompt you to start exercising religiously every single day? And if only, by following all the Pilates movements, you would immediately become awash in self-confidence and charm again! Unfortunately half the battle of feeling like a goddess again resides not in the body but in the mind. What we can do is alert you to a number of potential psychological obstacles to feeling good about your body and staying excited about working out. It is hard not to fall prey, at least temporarily, to some of these hurdles some of the time, but identifying and anticipating them can help you jump over them as quickly as possible.

Beware the "I'm too fat to work out" syndrome.   Far too many women can feel so defeated by the current state of their bodies that they cannot motivate themselves to begin any fitness program. It's as if any attempt at self-improvement feels pointless, so why even bother? This viewpoint couldn't be more wrong, of course. Every little bit counts in exercise. With PeeWee Pilates, just doing the minimal five-minute stomach series can build abdominal muscle tone. Besides, once you notice a slight improvement in your body, the change can become incredibly reinforcing and you will find yourself wanting to do more and more.

Calling yourself names doesn't help.   It can be tempting to tell yourself that the only reason why *you and you alone* look like crap five months after giving birth is because *you* are "out of control," "undisciplined," "lazy," or otherwise inadequate. Unfortunately, berating yourself won't give you the kick in the pants you need to exercise. On the contrary, indulging in these self-destructive assaults will only undermine your motivation to exercise and intensify your poor feelings about your body. Besides, you are not alone in how you feel about your body. It is incredibly common for women to feel dissatisfied with their bodies for at least a full year after giving birth.

Don't trivialize what you just went through.   Carrying a baby for nine months and going through childbirth were Herculean tasks! Do not play them down. Remind yourself of this miracle that your body just achieved, developing, housing, and nurturing new life. Consider the possibility that your pregnancy-related changes in physique are all part of your badge of honor for bringing a new person into the world. No exercise program, including Pilates, can guarantee to completely reverse the physical toll that pregnancy took on your body. Especially after multiple births, abdominal ligaments, pelvic floor muscles, and other body parts may continue forever to remind you of the essential job they once performed in bringing life to your baby. Bodies are not meant to look like the airbrushed mannequins you see in many magazines. What we would like to encourage you to do is redefine your maternal body based on the achievement it just pulled off. Wear your maternal badge proudly!

Cancel your membership in the "mothers are not supposed to be sexy" club. Motherhood does not have to be equated with giving up your own beauty and style. It is not just movie stars who are entitled to be simultaneously glamorous and maternal. Far too many women regress into frumpiness when they become mothers, putting all their energies instead into their children, perhaps guided by some unconscious belief that to be a good mother, you ought to cast aside your own physical pride and sexuality. Caring for yourself does not have to take anything away from your children. As described earlier, when we care for and feel good in our own bodies, we provide an important role model for our children. We should add here that you don't have to wait until you have lost every single pregnancy pound or firmed up your buttocks to feel sexy and attractive again. Far too many new mothers may avoid having sex with their partner because they feel too unappealing![17]

Don't despair just because your body doesn't bounce back like Gwyneth Paltrow's or Julia Roberts's. How reasonable are your expectations about your physical appearance? What kind of yardstick are you using to measure how thin or shapely or muscular you should be? Setting up unrealistic expectations for yourself can seriously undermine your efforts to eat healthfully and exercise, since you are far more likely to give up in frustration when your efforts fail to achieve the results you are aiming for.[18] Most of us women can't help but reflexively assess how good we look by comparing ourselves to other women around us. As a new mother, you may find yourself checking out the other moms in your "mommy and me" class or your pediatrician's office. Such ridiculous assessments can cause you a lot of unnecessary grief. The more you compare your own appearance to that of others, the more likely you are to perpetuate personal feelings of inferiority. Also, you need to be mindful of how you go about choosing a comparison group. Evaluating yourself against a woman who is fifteen years younger than you or a celebrity who has an in-house trainer and a personal chef is a recipe for disaster. You also need to take into account the fact that different women may be predisposed to respond to the physical aspects of pregnancy in very different ways. For example, it has been found that certain subgroups of women, especially African-American women, are more vulnerable to retaining weight in the postpartum period.[19] Women who are breast-feeding may also retain fat on their bodies differently from women who opt to bottle-feed. Some women may experience a slowdown in their metabolism after pregnancy, perhaps due to thyroid changes; for other women, it can seem as if their metabolism has gone into overdrive during the postpartum period and they can barely consume enough compensatory calories.

Don't let the mirror or scale be the sole arbiter of your attractiveness. Try to judge your body based on your internal sense of yourself rather than on how you compare yourself to others, what you think you see in the mirror, or the number that registers on the scale. Consider how your body *feels*, not just how it looks. Are you building muscle in your abdomen? Are you able to increase the reps on most of the exercises? Do you feel any more energetic or alert? Are you gaining strength in your limbs and middle? Does it feel any easier to stand up straight now, with your shoulders pressed back and your abdomen pulled in? Focusing on the function of your body, not just its appearance, can be a lot more rewarding. By following an exercise program such as yoga or Pilates, you can discover and strengthen muscle groups in your body that you never even knew were there.

Don't assume that others are always on flaw patrol.   Just because you may be self-conscious about how you look doesn't mean that others are regarding you with the same critical eye. Studies have shown that women who have a body image disturbance tend to overrate the degree to which others notice their physical attributes.[20] However, when you do come face to face with someone who does seem decidedly on flaw patrol, such as a parent or spouse, you may need to carefully consider where that person is coming from. Sometimes, a new mother needs to allow for the fact that she is not the only one who is adjusting to the changes in her maternal body. A husband may also miss your flat-as-a-board belly and may have feelings about your weight change or your swollen breasts. This is perfectly normal and doesn't mean he doesn't love you. Just as you need to go a little easy on yourself, you also may need to give him some slack—as long as he doesn't become overly critical or obnoxious.

Avoid declaring your appearance is either "all good" or "all bad."   This "all or nothing" thinking fails to take into account the fact that our presentation to the world is based on a composite of thousands of different personal physical features. These can include the lift of the neck, the fullness of the lips, a dimple in the cheek, the shape of the chin, broad shoulders, and so forth. To reduce your entire physical being to the category of "bad," based perhaps on carrying some extra pounds or possessing a flabby belly, is quite simply ridiculous. Try to consider a few attributes about yourself that you actually enjoy.

chapter 3

Wonderbaby

Understanding How Your Baby
Benefits from PeeWee Pilates

*"Even though you love your baby more than words can say, you will at
times look at him or her and think, 'You're just a blob!'"*

Jenny McCarthy,
*Belly Laughs: The Naked Truth About
the First Year of Mommyhood,* p. 109.

As you begin the exercises in PeeWee Pilates, you may question how in
the world your baby is possibly going to benefit from *your* workout.
After all, none of the movements require your baby to perform "spine
twists" or "leg kicks," let alone study flash cards or execute any major gym-
nastic feats. While you're toiling away, tucking, curling, squeezing, and lifting, your baby is just hanging out, making goo-goo eyes at you or lounging
around peacefully. What's in it for your baby, you might wonder, besides
having to contend with a sweaty mom?

You'd be surprised. Infant research has shown that right out of the starting gate, almost every aspect of a baby's brain is profoundly shaped by her

relationships with the primary caretakers in her life. As you work out to-gether with your baby—perhaps while holding her, singing, gazing, smiling, making faces, talking "baby talk," rocking, stroking, or otherwise consorting with your little one—you can dramatically stimulate your baby's emotional, intellectual, and motor growth. Your attentive interactions can enhance just about everything: her social skills, coping style, attention span, curiosity, memory, language development, sense of logic, intuition, physical agility, and even her mathematical abilities. While your baby is interacting with you, she is maximally motivated to "exercise" her own budding skills. She is so determined to grab and sustain your attention that, in your presence, she will experiment over and over again with efforts to hear, vocalize, move, smell, smile, and so on, all so that she can connect with you. As you respond to her communications, returning her coos, replying with your own silly faces, picking her up when she starts to cry, you are helping your baby to consolidate control of her own senses and growing competencies, and you are helping her to understand that her behavior has consequences. And that's just for starters.

PeeWee Pilates is an ideal forum for showering your baby with a full range of visual, tactile, auditory, and motor stimulation, all of which, as you will learn, can accelerate your baby's development. Each PeeWee Pilates exercise obliges you to engage in some kind of multisensory contact with your baby. More specifically:

1. Throughout most of the exercises, your baby is within inches of your face so that you can maintain direct, face-to-face contact. Gazing back and forth at each other is no idle sport; this mutual gaze between a mom and her baby provides a foundation for almost everything from your baby's social relatedness to his language proficiency.

2. Your baby is always within easy reach, so that you have lots of opportunity to spoil him with hugs, massage, and gentle caresses. Babies re-

spond dramatically to touch expressed in a loving, caring manner. For example, infants who are given frequent massages may actually have accelerated memory and sensory discrimination skills, abilities that are predictive of intellectual functioning years later.[1]

3. While your baby comes along for the ride as you progress through your exercises, he gets swung and rocked, which will delight his senses and treat him to a series of novel visual perspectives. Such movements stimulate your baby's vestibular system, a kind of "sixth sense" that enables your baby to perceive his body's balance and movement in space.[2] Stimulating your baby's vestibular system can significantly speed up the development of his reflexes, motor skills, and visual alertness.

4. As your baby accompanies you through the exercises, he will be encouraged to "practice" his developing motor skills, especially by being given lots of "tummy time." In tummy time, the small infant is placed in a position to push up on his arms in order to look around, see the world, and gain awareness of some of his muscles. Because you are literally on the floor with your baby, right at his level, you offer your baby a comfortable, safe environment that will encourage him to actively explore his own body and his motor skills.[3]

5. And of course, while you are hanging out with your baby, we strongly encourage you to deluge him with sounds; talk to him, sing, tell him about all the parts of the body that you are using, repeat syllables that you hear him emitting. The more you talk to your baby, the more his own language skills are likely to flourish.

Take note that we are *not* suggesting that you can override your baby's own internally wired developmental timeline. No amount of "teaching" or "coaxing" can manipulate a baby to do something for which he or she lacks neuromuscular readiness. When we talk about "stimulation," we mean providing opportunities that encourage your baby to discover how to organize his experience in the world. With this "practice," babies gain confidence, become more interested in performing a given activity, and seek out more efficient neural circuits to draw on.

Understanding Infant Development

A quick lesson on infant development will help explain how PeeWee Pilates provides such a good fit for your baby as you perform your own workout. As you read this chapter, your growing awareness of how much your interactions with your baby affect her development can only help you become a more sensitive, creative, resourceful partner to your baby, both during your workouts and throughout your day together.

Compared with other species, we humans come into this world with surprisingly "incomplete" or "immature" brains.[4] What this means exactly is that a significant portion of our actual brain development takes place *after* we are born. To give you some perspective, about 70 percent of the final DNA content of your baby's brain is not added until after birth.[5] And in the first year of life alone, your baby's brain will gain almost a pound and a half,[6] practically tripling in size.[7] Although genetics certainly plays a significant role in predetermining how your baby's brain will develop, her expanding brain is highly dependent upon her experiences, especially her interactions with the primary people in her life. To put it more precisely, your baby's close, early experiences literally sculpt her brain.

The brain is made up of a complex network of neurons, or nerve cells that are shaped like trees with ever-expanding roots, called dendrites. Every time your baby casts her eyes on an image, hears a sound, feels a touch, or has a thought, she is enlisting her brain power, and electrical activity is coursing through the neurons in her brain. Dendrites are stimulated to grow, and synapses (the connections between the neurons) form. In addition, myelin, a fatty substance, coats the nerve fibers, speeding up the transmission of electrical signals in the brain. In the first year of life, as your baby explores her own body and the fascinating new world around her, especially her fascinating mama, her brain is abuzz, processing all this new information by rapidly forming hundreds of thousands of new synapses and laying down elaborate neural circuits. Those synaptic connections that are used more frequently become increasingly strong and efficient. The exact refinement of this neural network hugely influences how your little girl's mind will work. It will determine how she'll make sense of what she sees in the world, how she'll relate to others, and how she'll think about herself. As your baby's brain wiring becomes more sophisticated, she becomes better equipped to understand and more skillfully engage with her environment; this success, in turn, promotes new learning experiences and more brain growth and enrichment. Clearly, our babies need rich interpersonal experience to flourish. Fortunately, as they go about their business of caring for their baby, most parents can't help but naturally provide heaps of loving stimulation. In the PeeWee Pilates exercises, you will have one more opportunity to be up close and personal with your baby, stimulating her brain while you're getting yourself in shape.

Emotions Rule!

When we talk about your baby interacting with you, we are referring most importantly to your *emotional* dialogue. In fact, there is a strong consensus across disciplines—from neurobiologists to psychoanalysts—that your baby's *emotional* attachment to you significantly organizes how his mind is constructed and how he will perceive and manage his emotional states. As the highly regarded pediatrician Dr. Stanley Greenspan puts it, "Emotions are actually the internal architects, conductors, or organizers of our minds. They tell us and show us what to think, what to say and when to say it, and what to do. We 'know' things through our emotional interactions and then apply that knowledge to the cognitive world." In fact, as Greenspan explains, the infant's emotional reactions are "giving each sensory experience texture and meaning."[8]

Your baby is an incredibly astute observer of emotions. Infants as young as four weeks old can register when you're in a good or bad mood! Between four and eight months of age, babies can also read some of your facial expressions and react positively or become upset depending upon what they see.[9] This doesn't mean that you have to appear cheerful every second of the day. In fact, infants can benefit when they are exposed to a variety of emotions.[10] But it does mean that you need to try to remain consistently sensitive to your baby's emotional needs, whether you're working out or changing diapers. One of the best ways to ensure that you will be a sensitive nurturer is to make sure that you nurture your own needs. When you enhance your own sense of well-being and calm, you can't help but become more relaxed, nurturing, and responsive with your baby.

What does it mean to be consistently sensitive to your baby's emotional needs anyway? First of all, it means being attuned to your baby's rapidly shifting moods and emotions. Babies can transition very rapidly from one emotional state to another in quick, fleeting bursts. To help you track these shifts, your baby communicates to you with a whole cache of nonverbal gestures and sounds. We're sure you're familiar with the bloodcurdling cry, pleading with you to "pay attention!" Other cues, however, may be somewhat more subtle to interpret, like a frown or a slight whimper or a turn of the head. Let's say you're entertaining your baby with a favorite rock, rap, or reggae tune. You rhythmically bounce her up and down to the beat of the music. Your daughter decides, however, that she is more in the mood for a soft lullaby; she begins to squirm and arch her back, and then she slowly builds up into a full-throttled cry. Don't take it personally! It doesn't mean you have a terrible voice or that she won't become a music lover. Babies strive toward an optimal level of arousal, and their moods can change as they try to strike this balance. If they are not sufficiently aroused, they may seek out more stimulation, perhaps by giving you one of their famous irresistible grins. If they are over-aroused, they may look away momentarily after you've been playing together for a while. It's as if they sometimes need a little cooling-off time to process the interaction before they are ready to go again. If they are negatively aroused, babies might need a hug, gentle stroking, or soft singing.

Once you read your baby's signals, it is important to respond promptly. This way, your baby develops an expectation that you will be there for him when he needs you and can enjoy a more secure attachment to you. He will learn that he can count on you to help him manage his own emotions, he will grasp the concept of cause and effect (he cries; you respond), and he will begin to learn how to regulate his own feelings.

Of course, no one expects you to be perfect. Don't feel that you need to respond to your baby's every little grimace or that you need to decipher perfectly every signal your baby emits. Misreading your child's signals, feelings, or needs is inevitable. In fact, falling out of sync and then reestablishing attunement can be an invaluable experience for your baby. When you are willing to recognize that you've made a mistake and try to fix it by redoubling your efforts, you offer your baby a powerful lesson. You're teaching him to hang in there during moments of frustration, and to have a kind of faith that misunderstandings can be overcome, that others care enough to repair potential hurts. This faith promotes enormous emotional resilience in your baby.[11]

Baby-Mama Drama

Communicating with your baby is not a one-way street. Without your probably even realizing it, you and your baby spend countless moments together engaging in an ongoing reciprocal communication dance. Your baby babbles to you and you vocalize back, trying to repeat or accentuate some of his sounds. He smiles and expectantly awaits your return smile; most of the time, you can't resist smiling back. He opens his mouth wide and watches you mirror back an exaggerated form of his expression. You then stick out your tongue and he does the same. What you may not realize is just how naturally you probably join in the "dance." You may raise the pitch of your voice, speak in a rising melody, and regress into baby talk as your baby shows increasing delight in your attention. Every gesture, touch, gaze, or vocalization that either of you makes in relation to one another is part of your conversation. The more expert your baby becomes at this back-and-forth interpersonal communication, the more likely it is that he will become a socially skilled, emotionally capable youngster.[12] Letting your baby take the lead in this dance especially encourages him to enjoy his own spontaneous expressions and develop confidence.

It is especially important as you communicate together that your own emotional level is in synchrony with your baby's emotional expression. When your baby is content, you reflect back joy; when he cries, your own mood becomes more subdued. Such moment-to-moment matching of emotions helps both you and your baby to feel more emotionally connected to one another. This emotional matching is so important that it can predict a great deal about how your baby will function months and years later. It can predict how he will cope with his emotional life and how readily he will develop language. The nature of the reciprocity between mother and baby can even predict how your baby will relate to his peers and perform in school many years later.[13]

Encourage Your Baby to Exercise Her Senses!

Right from birth, your baby draws on all of her sensory systems (vision, hearing, movement, sensation, and touch) to perceive and begin to understand her world. If you're nursing your baby, for example, she is having a multisensory experience of you: She tastes your milk, smells your body, gazes into your face, and feels the texture of your skin against hers. The more skilled your baby is at coordinating and integrating all her varied senses, the more resilient and adaptable she is likely to be.

According to Esther Thelen, a well-regarded developmental psychologist:

> Every waking moment includes sensations not only from vision, hearing, taste, smell, and feeling but also from receptors in muscles, joints, and skin that detect position, force, and movement changes in a continually active organism. What is important is that the nervous system is built to integrate these streams of information: The senses are richly interconnected between and among many anatomically distinct areas. . . . It may be exactly this continual bombardment of real-life, multi-sensory but coherent information that fuels the engines of developmental change as infants learn to act in social and physical worlds.[14]

As you bounce, lift, and rock your own baby, you are bombarding her with a rich variety of sensory information.

Let's look at the different senses through which your baby comes to understand her world and communicates with you. As you perform PeeWee Pilates, you will want to pay attention to how you can optimally engage your baby's different senses. You will want to observe just how your baby takes you in and seeks you out using everything she's got: her eyes, skin, ears, smiles, cute little coos, and piercing cries. Each baby, of course, has her own highly personal, idiosyncratic way of responding to the world. As you spend time with your own infant, you will get to know her particular preferences. Some babies long for exciting, loud stimulation and are thrilled by flashing lights, daring swings in the air, or even a loud drum roll. Other babies, on the contrary, can become easily overstimulated; a gentle touch can feel too ticklish, and an excited laugh can become noxious. Babies also differ in their overall activity level; some babies are nonstop wiggle worms, and other babies are content to serenely contemplate their surroundings. Babies also vary in their willingness to explore new tastes, sounds, and sights. Some babies become downright ornery when presented with a novel sound until they have a chance to acclimate. Other babies thrive on the excitement of a new discovery. It is important to learn to pay attention to—and respect—your own baby's temperament, sensory preferences, and moment-to-moment shifts in desire.

Here's Looking at You!

Some people believe that vision is the most important of all the senses because it helps your baby synthesize everything he hears, tastes, smells, and feels as he moves about his world.[15] Surprisingly, however, babies are born with very poor vision. As a newborn, your baby can only see about eight inches in front of him, and the images that he can perceive are blurry at best and lack a range of color. With experience, however, the part of your baby's brain that is involved in vision, his visual cortex, will develop very rapidly, and by his six-month-old checkup, he will develop depth perception, reasonable acuity, controlled eye movements, and color perception.[16] By about one year old, your baby's vision will be almost on par with an adult's.

So how can you stimulate your baby's vision? As you may already know from all the infant toys on the market, your young infant is drawn to bold objects and patterns, black-and-white contrasts, and slow-moving objects. If you want to attract his attention, offer slowly rotating monochromatic objects, like a black-and-white mobile. But you also have something else readily at your disposal that your baby loves to look at, and that is you, or really your *face*. Despite your baby's immature vision, straight from birth he is prewired to prefer faces over any other visual image. In fact, it has been suggested that babies are born with an ability (referred to as a *face-detecting device*) to zero in on features and to recognize that a face is in fact a face and not some inanimate blob. You might be interested to know that babies prefer to look at "attractive" faces, but their version of attractive is not necessarily in keeping with that of *Vogue* magazine. Babies prefer faces that have readily classifiable facial features, like big eyes, distinctive noses, and so on.[17] Regardless of how attractive you feel yourself to be, do not worry; in the long run, your baby will still prefer to look at your face over any other. In fact, within a few hours after birth, he can already distinguish your face from those of other women. If your baby is younger than two months old, he will prefer to look at your face if it's moving slowly.[18] After two months, you can still catch his attention without moving your head. Just seeing your face can be enough to stop a two-month-old baby from crying—sometimes!

By your baby's third month, he doesn't just want to peer at your face. He wants to look into your eyes and engage you in brief one- or two-minute face-to-face animated interactions. Mothers seem to know this instinctually because they tend to present their faces in full view of their infants to encourage eye-to-eye contact. Babies can respond to even very subtle shifts in the adult's eye gaze. A series of well-known research studies referred to as the *still-face experiments* painfully illustrates how upset babies can become when denied eye contact and responsive facial feedback.[19] In the experiments, three- or four-month-old babies looked at their mothers, trying to communicate with them, but the mothers were instructed to remain unexpressive. Infant after infant increased his attempts to connect with the mother. Then, when these infants' repeated efforts were unsuccessful, they began to protest and then became agitated and disorganized.

It turns out that when your baby has eye contact with you, he not only can gaze into your eyes but can also learn to follow your gaze. Following your gaze allows your baby to check out what you're looking at (when you're not looking right at your little cutie) and to figure out what you think is so interesting. Babies who are more skilled at following a parent's eye gaze at six months of age have actually been found to have a larger vocabulary a year and a half later. Researchers have explained that if you look where your mom is looking, maybe you can figure out what she is talking about when she uses words.[20] While you are working out with your baby, you might play with the idea of watching your baby track your gaze. See if he turns his head to look where you're looking. (Don't worry, however, if your baby cannot master this for a while; different babies develop this skill at different rates, often not until well after nine months of age.)

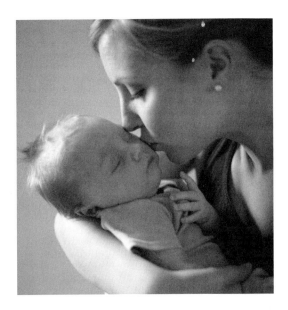

The Magic Touch

No one has to tell you just how wonderful it can be to embrace your soft, cuddly baby and delight in the pure silky feel of her skin. In fact, you were prewired to find your baby irresistible, with good reason. Physical contact with one's mother (or another primary caretaker) is a basic need of all babies; without it, babies simply cannot flourish. The sheer act of touching your baby can have a surprisingly huge impact on her actual physical growth as well as on her emotional, intellectual, and physical adaptation.

Why is touch such a big deal? Touch offers your baby a tangible, reassuring message that you are solidly present. Enveloped in your safe, containing embrace, your baby can feel secure enough to check out the world around her, knowing that she is protected by you. Touch can also be incredibly soothing. Of course, this is not earth-shattering news to you. When your baby cries, you pick her up and hold her against you, and her distress usually diminishes. What you might not be aware of, however, is that when babies are soothingly stroked or massaged, they have been shown to exhibit a drop in their cortisol levels (a chemical that measures the bodily experience of stress). Remember, too, that cuddling can produce oxytocin, a hormone that promotes feelings of calm and affection. Touch is inherently an incredibly intimate, nurturing human interaction that facilitates feelings of attachment. How you exchange touch with your baby will deeply shape her feelings about herself and the world around her. When you regularly touch your baby in a sensitive, warm manner, you help lay a foundation for her relationships in the future, where she can come to rely upon and enjoy warm, intimate involvements with others. Interestingly, how often you touch your baby can also help *you* to feel more emotionally attached to your little person.[21]

In recent years, infant massage classes have become quite trendy, and their popularity is well deserved. A daily gentle massage that entails rubbing and stroking (but no tickling, which can cause adverse effects!) can improve your baby's functioning in many surprising ways. Regular massage can improve your infant's sleep, decrease her irritability, improve her sociability,[22] and even possibly promote the release of growth hormones.[23] Massage may also improve your baby's responsiveness to learning opportunities. In one study, four-month-old babies could actually learn something more quickly when they were given an eight-minute massage beforehand. Because of its effectiveness in accelerating infant growth as well as enhancing the mother-baby bond, infant massage has become a standard form of care for hospitalized premature babies. With daily massage, these babies can accelerate their development and often hasten their departure from the hospital.

Gee, Your Hair Smells Terrific!

Months before your baby even entered the world, he was busy developing and using his sense of smell. While he was in your womb, he was already responding to the aroma wafting from your kitchen (or your take-out bag), your perfume, and your shampoos. Within hours of his birth, your baby can pick out your unique bodily scent or the smell of your breast milk.[24] This is a two-way street. You, too, can identify your own baby by his smell alone almost immediately after birth. Even if you haven't showered, no matter how stinky you are, your own scent can be extremely comforting to your baby. Babies as little as three days old may calm down their movements when they are in contact with your smell.[25] In fact, smell plays an essential role in maternal-infant bonding. The mutual attraction to each other's pheromones strengthens your already intense bond. While you're working out, your body odor can actually be quite pleasing and even enticing to your baby—even if it keeps others away.

Someone's Listening!!

From the moment of birth, babies are actively listening to the world around them. In fact, of all the newborn's senses, hearing is one of the most well developed. During your last trimester of pregnancy, while you were lugging your baby around getting ready for labor, your baby was already busy developing her auditory skills. She had lots of opportunity in the womb to familiarize herself with your voice and listen to you read aloud and croon to her with your favorite songs. As soon as she was born, she could therefore already distinguish your voice from other women's voices, prefer the language which she heard you speak during the last trimester of your pregnancy, and show a preference for those songs or stories she actually "remembered" from the good old days in your belly. You may have noticed that your baby is now so responsive to your voice that she will move her body in synchrony with the rhythm of your speech. Just be sure that you turn up the volume ever so slightly. Newborns cannot hear especially soft, quiet sounds and even by six months of age are still a little hard of hearing.

Your baby is an attentive, discriminating, appreciative listener. She can enjoy the complexity of classical music (though the alleged "Mozart effect" has been found to be completely overrated in terms of its ability to turn your baby into a genius)[26] as well as the soothing, calming quality of a sweet lullaby. Astoundingly subtle differences in sounds, especially the sounds of speech, do not escape the notice of your keen little listener. Young infants can discriminate nearly every type of speech sound—or phoneme—that exists and are ready to learn any language in the world to which they're exposed. By just four and a half months of age, your baby can find the cues to figure out where one sentence ends and the next one begins just by listening to the melody of language.

Certain sounds are more likely to capture your baby's attention. Babies prefer higher-pitched voices with exaggerated singsong intonations and a slightly slower tempo. As it turns out, this is exactly what characterizes baby talk or "motherese"—or to be more politically correct, "parentese." When you speak baby talk to your little one, she is much more likely to pay attention; it's as if she realizes that this special kind of speech is meant exclusively for her. Speaking in an adult tone just won't grab your baby's attention as effectively. At just about four months of age, your baby can also recognize her name. (You can test this out by calling your baby's name—or better yet, having someone your baby does not know call her name—and see if your baby perks up.)[27] Once your baby learns that she is Zoe or Isabel or whatever name she is connected to, she can begin to discover the symbolic power of language. Hearing her name will also draw her attention to the words that come together with it. For example, if you say, "Kai, want a banana?" pairing the word *banana* with your baby's name will help your baby master the words *want* and *banana* more quickly. In this way, from about four months to seven and a half months of age, babies use their names as an "anchor" to help decipher speech patterns. Most of you mothers know all this intuitively and do this quite effortlessly; you tend to repeat your baby's name often, and you easily regress into high-pitched, baby talk.

Can We Please Talk?

Babies aren't just content to hang around like bystanders, listening to you do all the talking. They want a piece of the action. They want to share in animated conversations with you. Long before your baby can articulate a single word, he will emit all sorts of sounds, from cries of hunger to shrieks of joy to contented cooing, all in an effort to communicate with you. How you respond to his efforts will have a huge impact not only on your baby's language skills but also on his overall intellectual, social, and emotional development. According to Lise Eliot, author of *What's Going On in There? How the Brain and Mind Develop in the First Five Years of Life*, "Speech is without doubt the most important form of stimulation a baby receives. When parents talk to their babies they are activating hearing, social, emotional, and linguistic centers of the brain all at once, but their influence on language development is especially profound."[28] Study after study has found that mothers who vocalize with their babies in a reciprocal, responsive fashion tend to have smarter, more verbally skilled babies.[29] In one study, the quantity and quality of mothers' conversations with their infants during a home visit directly predicted their child's level of intelligence as many as twelve years later.[30]

How do your conversations with your baby encourage him to speak?

- Babies love to connect emotionally with you. When you engage your baby in direct, focused conversation, facing him and matching the cadence of his own speech or breath with your speech, your baby will often be eager to reciprocate by vocalizing right back to you.

- Babies love to imitate what they hear. Starting at two months of age, infants will try to match the pitch of their parent's voice. If you speak right after your baby has emitted a sound, your baby is likely to reply back with sounds that more closely approximate real speech.[31]
- As your baby listens to you talk, his brain is attending to every sound you produce, that is, all those vowels and consonants you speak in your own native tongue. All the sounds that your baby hears shape his neural circuits and prepare him to begin talking.
- When you talk with your baby, you also teach him the fundamentals of taking turns. While your baby communicates, you stop and listen. When he pauses, you offer your reply.

Your baby's most obvious and earliest means of conversing with you is by crying. Crying is your baby's signal to you that he needs your attention. There are actually many different kinds of cries, varying in level of pitch depending upon the emotions they convey. Though you may not even realize it, you decipher these different cries all the time. For example, you can intuit whether your baby is crying because he's hungry, is in some kind of pain, or because he is overwhelmed by some unpleasant stimuli.

Between one and three months, your baby begins to play more happily with sounds. First, he entertains you with cooing, those charming "oooohs" and "aaaahs" that tell you that your baby is feeling quite content and is eager to converse with you. Between six and ten months of age, your baby's vocalizations progress to babbling, which is characterized by the repetition of consonants and vowels. As your baby produces all these different sounds, he is developing the muscles in his mouth, throat, lips, and so on, as well as his neuromotor circuitry. As you respond to his cooing and babbling (which, again, no one expects you to do *all the time;* the average mother only responds to these vocalizations about 35 percent of the time),[32] you can offer finely tuned responses by pausing briefly to listen to your baby talk, imitate his own sounds, and emit high-pitched vocalizations with rising melodies.[33]

Moving

Your baby craves motion! While she may not yet be ready to tackle the triple-loop roller coaster, for her, repetitive bouncing, spinning, and rocking in your arms is the perfect amusement park. As you swing, rock, or bounce your baby, the motion alters the fluid in her inner ear; this sensory input, called vestibular stimulation, informs her brain about the orientation or position of her body in space. We all rely upon our vestibular system to help us maintain balance and head and body posture as we move about in the world. Basically, the way that it works is that tiny hair cells in and around the inner ear move around as they perceive shifts in our balance and movement. This movement of the hair cells then elicits messages to special vestibular neurons, which in turn send messages to the brain and the spinal cord about how our body is moving and positioned in space. Vestibular stimulation seems to have a calming, organizing effect on babies,[34] but you probably already know this because when your baby is fussy, irritable, or tense, it is second nature to pick her up and gently jiggle her while you walk around the room. Surprisingly, comforting a crying baby by rocking or bouncing her can have the unexpected side effect of improving her visual alertness, which in turn, can help her pay keener attention to her surrounding environment. Vestibular stimulation, according to Eliot, can also dramatically accelerate the development of your baby's reflexes and motor skills, such as her head control, sitting, crawling, and walking.

What a spectacular transformation your baby's motor skills undergo in the span of just one short year of life! She comes into this world unable to hold her head up or roll over on her side, and yet, just one year later (give or take a few months), she can strut independently right across your living room floor and get into so many things that you'd better start baby-proofing your home! How does your baby pull this off? The answer, mostly, is genetics. Thanks to biological programming, healthy babies from such diverse places as Bombay, Dublin, and New York City all learn to sit and crawl and grasp objects with just their thumb and forefinger in the same exact sequence at the exact same age (give or take just a couple of months). However, if motor development were exclusively shaped by genes, your baby's interactions with her environment would have absolutely no bearing on her capacity to learn a new task or grasp a new concept. In the last decade or two, researchers and clinicians have begun to determine that this is simply not the case. They have discovered that some experiences during infancy definitely matter, but not necessarily as we might expect. Your baby's motor skills develop as a "continual dialogue between the nervous system, body, and environment."[35] What this means is that although you can't teach your baby how to crawl, sit, or reach *before* these capabilities are ready to emerge on their own, you can inundate your baby with motion, which can, in turn, stimulate her vestibular system, expand her range of movement, and accelerate the growth of her motor skills. You can also encourage your baby to "practice" the motor skills that she has already begun to exhibit. By providing your baby with (1) a comfortable, open area to move about and explore, (2) patient, nearby support, and (3) a gentle nudge to practice a move when she is "just on the cusp of acquiring each skill,"[36] you can encourage your baby to make the most of her emerging capabilities at any given time. Left to her own devices, your baby is naturally quite motivated to repeatedly perform the newest body movements that she has learned. Babies like to give themselves homework assignments such as "Work on crawling."[37]

Babies learn best when they are the initiators of their own movements and explorations.[38] When babies generate their own movements, they discover that they can cause interesting consequences. Recognizing that they can cause something to happen is very reinforcing; they will want to do this over and over again. For example, in a simple, ingenious series of experiments, a mobile was connected to a baby's foot with a ribbon; whenever the baby kicked that foot, the mobile would begin to rotate. As babies quickly figured out that their kicking accelerated the spinning of the mobile, they would kick more and more vigorously. In this way, they demonstrated a capability for planned or volitional action.[39]

As your baby gains confidence in her ability to move about on her own, she will become increasingly eager to explore her environment. In turn, the more she explores, the more she will learn about the physical properties of her world. As Esther Thelen wrote, "It is only by moving eyes and head, hands and arms, and traveling from one place to another that people can fully experience the environment and learn to adapt to it. During development, then, each motor milestone opens new opportunities for perceptual discovery."[40]

What difference does it make how quickly your child achieves different motor skills? What if your baby is one of those kids who are reluctant to sit up or crawl? First of all, resist the impulse to obsessively compare what your own little one is doing in relation to the other babies around you. As long as your baby achieves significant milestones like sitting and grasping within about two or three months of the so-called average baby, she falls squarely within the "normal" range of development. The age at which your baby's different motor skills emerge says nothing at all about your child's overall intellectual level. What is much more important is how your baby relates to you and how she is developing her capacity to use all her senses in an integrated, coordinated fashion.

In Chapter 6, you will learn more about how to apply this information as you engage with your baby throughout the PeeWee Pilates exercises.

Part II

Getting Started

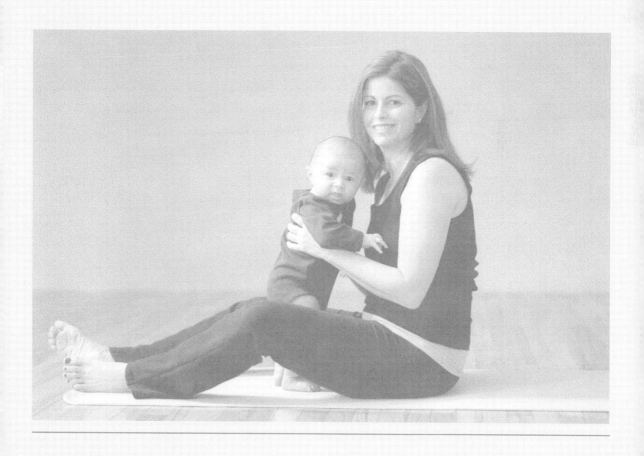

Roll out your mat! You're almost ready to start your workout.

Before you begin, we'd like to go over a few basic exercise guidelines for postpartum women. Based on our consultation with a licensed obstetrician-gynecologist, there are a few areas of caution and concern that you may need to keep in mind as you go about your workout. We also want to acquaint you with some of the principles and foundations of Pilates for those of you who are not already familiar with this method. Those of you who are fluent in Pilates-speak may still find it helpful to review this section, especially since you're adding your baby to the picture. The better prepared you are, the easier it will be to follow the exercises. These instructions will also help ensure a safe, productive, and satisfying workout.

In the next three chapters, you will find all the information you need to get started with your workout. In Chapter 4, we will give you all the basics about getting started, when you can begin, some contraindications you need to consider, and what you need to have on hand. In Chapter 5, you will receive a crash course in the basics of Pilates. Be sure not to miss Chapter 6, which will give you lots of helpful information about how to turn your baby into the ideal exercise partner.

chapter 4

Roll Out Your Mat!

*"You control more than 70 percent of how well
and how long you live . . ."*

Michael F. Roizen and Mehmet C. Oz,
You: The Owner's Manual, Harper Resource, 2005

Here are some basic suggestions to guide your workout. Please note, however, that these are only our recommendations. Consider them along with your own personal assessment of your postpartum condition, your fitness history, and your current needs. We have found that many women have a clear sense of what works best for their own bodies. Most women can tell when they're ready to get started, how hard to push themselves, and what the limits are of their own comfort threshold. Of course, checking in with your own physician about your own postpartum recovery status and readiness should supersede our suggestions. As a general rule, whenever you are in doubt, it is always best to ask your doctor.

"How Soon Is Now?" Starting PeeWee Pilates

If you had an uncomplicated vaginal delivery, you can start doing PeeWee Pilates as early as three to six weeks after giving birth. By starting, however, we don't mean jumping in headfirst. We mean starting slowly and cautiously. The six-week mark coincides with the time it takes for your uterus to become completely involuted, or shrunk back to its prepregnancy size.

If you had a cesarean section delivery, your starting date is another story. At your two-week visit, your doctor should be able to determine whether your scar is healing properly and if you are at risk for infection or wound separation. After your six-week checkup, as long as you are given the green light, you can begin PeeWee Pilates. Most women who have undergone a C-section prefer to follow the C-section modifications that we have outlined with each exercise. However, for those of you who are feeling more energetic and confident about your recovery, feel free to try the regular exercises.

Proceed with Caution!

Unfortunately, there are a few medical conditions that may be serious enough to warrant postponing your PeeWee Pilates workout. These conditions all require full recovery and/or clearance from your doctor before you get started. Some of these concerns include:

- Severe complications from an episiotomy
- Postpartum bleeding: Occasional spotting or light bleeding is common and not something that need slow you down. What you don't want is clotting or heavy bleeding. If you experience heavy vaginal bleeding after a workout, then you probably have overdone it and may need to stop or slow down. Report to your doctor, especially if you have a fever, to rule out infection.
- High blood pressure: Some women can develop a condition during pregnancy called pregnancy-induced hypertension (PIH), which can

last for about six weeks after giving birth. It is essential that you get permission from your doctor before working out if you have been diagnosed with PIH.

Additional Speed Bumps

In the early stages of postpartum recovery, bear in mind that some possible conditions may arise that may need to be considered in your workout. None of these factors should stop you from working out, but they do call for a more cautious exercise approach.

1. **Joint laxity.** For a few months postpartum, you remain at risk for both overstretching and detaching your ligaments and developing instability in your joints. As explained in Chapter 1, the hormone relaxin stays in your body for about three months. One result is that the looseness in your joints can give you the false sense that you have a greater range of movement and flexibility than your frame really permits. Consequently, you may be tempted to overstretch and perform exaggerated, impulsive movements. Therefore it is important not to jump too quickly or too aggressively into any postpartum exercise program. Minor injuries from an overzealous workout may include sprains, muscle pulls, a pinched nerve, sciatica, and sacroiliac pain as well as a prolapsed bladder or uterus.

2. **Diastasis.** Many women develop a condition called diastasis recti. This is when a section of connective tissue between the longitudinal abdominal muscles weakens; the result is a small separation extending all the way down from your ribs to your pubic bone. You can detect this condition by running your finger straight down the midline of your body while lying on your back with your head tilted up. This

separation will often heal on its own, but you can accelerate healing by engaging specific muscles to encourage a narrowing of the split. See page 87.

3. **Hemorrhoids.** You may want to avoid certain exercises that involve sitting or rolling on your bottom if you are experiencing considerable discomfort.

Setting Up Shop:
What You Need on Hand to Get Started

Where: Just enough room to accommodate the length of your body plus about an extra foot on either side with room to spread your arms out full length. Create a relaxing, intimate atmosphere for you and your baby. Turn on the answering machine. Turn off the TV. Play music if you like. (Babies can be very responsive to rhythm and melody.)

Gear:
- *A padded gym mat* that can protect your spine throughout your workout. Make sure the padding is thick enough, at least one-half inch in depth. A yoga style mat may not give you enough cushioned protection from a hard floor. If you opt to use a yoga mat, you should fold it over so that the padding runs at least the length of your spine. Otherwise, a thick, soft blanket, folded over, can suffice, preferably placed on top of a soft carpet or rug for additional padding.
- *Two ample-sized, cushy blankets* (yoga blankets are preferred)
- A *small towel* (for baby messes, foot exercise, etc.)
- A *bottle of water.* Although it's always important to keep hydrated while exercising, it is paramount for postpartum women, especially those who are nursing.

Optional Gear:
- Yoga strap or exercise band
- Pillow
- Toys
- Hypoallergenic massage lotion or oil for baby
- Baby bottle
- Pacifier

Attire: For you, choose clothing in which you can move about easily. Take off your shoes. Socks are fine, though not necessary. Don't wear hanging jewelry. Your hair should be pulled back or away from your face.

Dress your baby in a simple onesy or other comfortable clothing that does not bunch up or hang in the way.

Approaching Your Workout

Take a moment to consider how you wish to approach your PeeWee Pilates workout. How motivated are you? How much time do you intend to give to your workouts? What kind of shape are you in *right now*? It is important to assess yourself realistically, taking into account the fact that your body is still recovering from a nine-month-long-ordeal and that your lifestyle now has dramatically changed. If you set up fitness expectations that you cannot possibly live up to because of limited time, exhaustion, weakness, or injury from your pregnancy, you are setting yourself up for failure. Establishing moderate, attainable exercise goals is essential to maintaining a workout routine for the long haul.[1] Many new mothers become easily discouraged when they encounter unexpected muscle weakness or fatigue or do not see results as quickly as they would like. Even if you were an Olympic athlete in tip-top shape before you got pregnant or you were one of those women who performed Pilates right through your pregnancy, you may discover that it is now slower going than you ever would have anticipated. However, with patience and a little self-discipline, you will regain strength quickly. Focus on using good form and don't force yourself to the point of strain. If you do get discouraged, hopefully the pleasure that you see registered in your baby's face during your workouts will persuade you to persist.

If, on the other hand, you find that the exercises seem too simple, you may not be doing them correctly. Remember that these exercises are quite subtle. Form is everything. The most seemingly straightforward movements may require a slight shift in positioning and focus. Don't rush yourself.

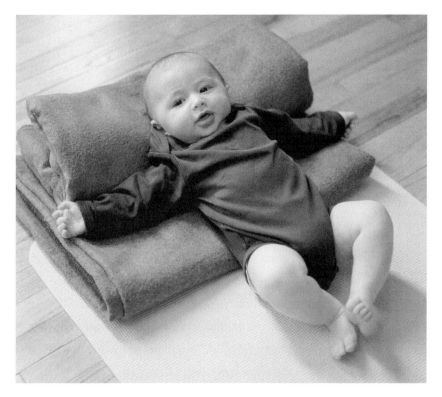

A nice way to prop up your baby using two blankets.

chapter 5

A Crash Course in Pilates

"Physical fitness is the first requisite of happiness."

———————

Joseph Pilates,
Pilates' Return to Life Through Contrology,
Presentation Dynamics, 1998

Pilates is not just the exercise mode du jour, waiting to be replaced by whatever new fitness craze comes next. The Pilates Method has been around for almost a full century. It was developed in Germany by Joseph Pilates, first as a means to fortify his own sickly body and later as a technique to accelerate the healing process for disabled soldiers. Since the 1920s, when Joseph Pilates immigrated to the United States and opened up his first Pilates studio, the Pilates method has attracted actors, dancers, football players, skaters, and other professional athletes, who rely significantly on their bodies for their work. In the last twenty years, Pilates has become a staple of millions of people's weekly fitness regimen.

Pilates is a full-body, vigorous workout comprising exercises that emphasize deep, slow, purposeful movements. These movements, which progress through specific body postures, demand intense muscle control. Most of the exercises consist of an alternating contraction and extension or stretching of the muscles in your body. When this alternating muscle action is executed in unison with proper breathing, the movements improve flexibility, build strength in your core, protect the joints, and reduce compression in the spine. A flexible, decompressed, elongated spine cannot be overrated. It offers a pillar of support for your entire body. Just for starters, it allows you to stand taller, feel better balanced, give your lungs space to breathe, and improve blood flow to your joints. However, the spine needs some assistance to stay erect, aligned, balanced, and stable. Enter the powerhouse. All of the Pilates movements are designed to add strength to what Pilates referred to affectionately as your core, or *powerhouse*. A strong powerhouse functions like a perfect-fitting corset; it supports your spine as well as the entire midsection of your body, including your important internal organs, by encasing and holding your middle together. Building strength in the powerhouse is considered the most important goal in Pilates. And right now *your* powerhouse might feel as if it has crossed the border for an extended vacation in Mexico. Well, the siesta is over, ladies!

We would like to familiarize you with some of the basic rules of Pilates. Make sure to keep these principles in mind as you move through your workouts.

The Nine Commandments of Pilates

First Commandment: Work from the Powerhouse!

This means that you are to work with intention from the middle of your body, not from your arms and legs. How do you know if you're working from the powerhouse? Ask yourself, "Is my lower back arching? Are my ribs sticking out? Are my shoulders hiking up toward my ears?" If you answer yes to any of these, you are probably not engaging your core and are putting yourself at risk for injury.

Second Commandment: Engage Your C Curve!

In the scoop position, or C curve, your navel is pulled back toward your spine, and your tailbone and pelvis are pulled under. Think of making the shape of the letter *C* with your body, starting at your tailbone and extending up to your mid back. Like the letter *C*, try to hollow or scoop out the front of your torso. Check yourself: If it feels as if you are constantly trying to pull your stomach away from your waistband, you are probably doing it correctly. This C curve opens up and articulates your spine.

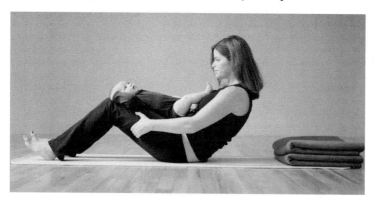

Third Commandment: Assume the Pilates Stance!

In simple terms, the Pilates stance is "heels together, toes apart." In this position, your legs should turn out slightly. Make sure not to rotate from your knees or ankles; the turnout should come naturally from the hip rotators to encourage deeper engagement from the pelvic floor. The inner thighs should pull forward as if the muscles are wrapping around the front of the thighs. Think about your legs resembling a Greek column. Do not try to emulate first position in ballet; that's too much turn out for the common gal.

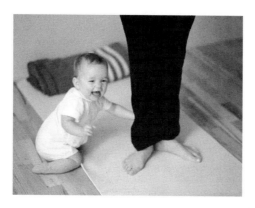

Fourth Commandment: Articulate Your Spine!

To articulate the spine is to roll up or down on your spine one vertebra at a time. Rolling fluidly and placing each vertebra distinctively onto the mat develops flexibility and elongation in the spine. For example, the Roll-Up and the Teaser, two movements that require you to roll up and down one vertebra at a time, allow you to release tension and elongate your spine while simultaneously strengthening your powerhouse. When you roll down on your spine, do you feel as if you're massaging your back, or do you hear a "thunk"? If it's the latter, your spinal column may be starting to compress, and you are at risk for stiffness, limited mobility, and poor circulation.

Fifth Commandment: Work Within Your Frame

When you move your body in proper alignment, you are essentially *working within the frame of your own body*, that is, within the width of your shoulders and hips. Precise movements that respect the structure and limits of your own body frame protect your joints from injury and promote healing. If you hear a pop or crack in a joint as you move, especially in the hips or shoulders, this may be a signal that you are working outside your frame. Joseph Pilates couldn't emphasize alignment enough! To ensure that good form and alignment are absolutely preserved with each movement, he insisted that each exercise be repeated no more than ten times. Maintaining alignment requires such effort and concentration that Joe Pilates believed it cannot be sustained during too many repetitions. As he liked to say, it is better to do ten perfect repetitions than fifty in poor form.

Sixth Commandment: Chin to the Chest

You'll see this instruction in many of the exercises. Quite plainly, it means lifting your head forward off the mat so that the back of your entire neck stretches and the chin reaches down into the chest area. Your gaze should be down toward the belly button. We do this to encourage the energy exerted to come from the powerhouse and create more space from the shoulders to the ears. Two questions you might ask yourself are: Am I looking up at the ceiling? Are my shoulders shrugged up to my ears? If you're holding your neck incorrectly, you can create tension in the neck and shoulders and possibly cause the lower back to arch off the mat.

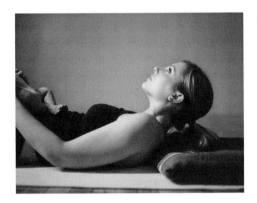 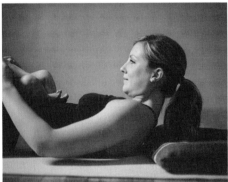

Seventh Commandment: Don't Be a Mouth Breather

Two simple rules here:

1. As Joseph Pilates used to say, "You eat with your mouth and breathe with your nose." Pilates breathing consists of both inhaling and exhaling audibly through your nose, taking slow deep breaths (in yoga this is referred to as *Ujjâyi*, or "victorious" breath). Your mouth stays out of the whole affair. Unlike the shallow breathing that results from respiration through the mouth, breathing through your nose enables you to fill your lungs to capacity and take in that much more oxygen.
2. Each breath in Pilates should be coordinated with your movement. Think of your body as an accordion. As you extend or expand, you inhale, pulling oxygen into the elongating muscles. As you contract

or bend inwards, you exhale, pushing out stale air. The deeper you breathe as you move through these exercises, the greater the benefits you will achieve. Proper breathing will discourage unnecessary muscle tension, which is so common to weight training and can cause stress-related injuries. This "victorious" breathing also encourages concentration and calm execution, which brings us to the next commandment.

Eighth Commandment: Move with Intention

Each exercise should be performed in a calm and focused manner. Don't throw yourself around like a whirling dervish. Since you only do up to ten repetitions of any one exercise at a time, try to maintain the integrity of your alignment. Make it worth your while by concentrating on moving slowly and deliberately. Don't force or rush through your exercises. Think *elegant!*

Ninth Commandment: No Powerhouse Was Built in a Day

Pilates is based on the principle of "adding on," that is, slowly adding exercises to your workout so that you build up to longer workouts. In other words, one never advances from the basic exercises that one starts with. You just add on a string of exercises to make your workout more demanding. Start slowly. You don't need to tackle everything in one day. If you master three to five exercises over the course of ten minutes each day, especially in the first few weeks of exercising, you're making good headway. Once you feel confident, challenge yourself by adding one or two new exercises.

Don't think that just because you're not sweating profusely or grunting through a thousand crunches you're not producing results. If you are a Pilates or yoga diva or you're very used to a more aggressive workout, you can probably tackle more exercises and repetitions for a longer period of time (going up to thirty to forty-five minutes).

Pilates and Yoga: A Perfect Partnership

Some people think of Pilates as a cross between yoga and calisthenics. In fact, Joseph Pilates based many of the exercises on traditional yoga asana. Although Pilates is a perfect complement to yoga, it can also take yoga to the next level, and vice versa. Therefore, we have decided to incorporate a few yoga-like postures in the last section of the exercises ("Aches, Pains, and Other Mommy Woes: Remedies Beyond PeeWee Pilates") to boost your total body workout. We also encourage you to pursue a yoga program in tandem with PeeWee Pilates, either on your own or in a mother-baby team, such as the Baby Om method.

How exactly do yoga and Pilates compare? Yoga (asana) asks you to hold a still posture for a period of time measured in breaths or minutes, depending upon the style of yoga that you practice. Pilates injects motion into postures. By building on these postures through movement, Pilates encourages core-strength building, balance, and an overall greater challenge to the abdominal muscles. A strong center can help you to avoid injury while practicing yoga, which can be deceptively challenging. In turn, yoga encourages deeper, more concentrated movement, breathing, and relaxation while also enhancing flexibility. Therefore, when you practice yoga, Pilates movements can become more accessible.

Many of the basic postures in Pilates will be familiar to the yoga practitioner. For example, the "plank position" in yoga shows up as the "leg pull down" in Pilates, and the "sphinx" in yoga closely resembles the Pilates "single leg kick." Similarly the focus on strengthening and articulating the powerhouse in Pilates is equally embraced in yoga, although the terminology and concept behind it are a bit different. In yoga, the powerhouse would be likened to the three "bandhas," or yoga locks ("organs or parts of the body that are contracted and controlled.")[1] The root lock, the mûla-bandha, entails squeezing the pelvic floor. The second lock is the uddîyâna-bandha, which entails pulling the navel to the spine and contracting the ribs. The third lock is the jâlandhara-bandha, which is a chin lock; in Pilates-speak, this is the "chin to the chest" head position.

Even the breathing is similar. In yoga, there are many different types of breathing (prânâyâma); the breath is in fact quintessential to yoga practice. Yogis refer to audible breathing through the nose, the same breath used in Pilates, as ujjâyi breathing. For yogis, ujjâyi breathing is used throughout asana practice to calm the mind and cleanse the system. Other breath techniques are also used in yoga to serve more specific functions; for example, kapâlabhâti (or shining skull breath) is done in rounds to clear one's sinuses. B. K. S. Iyengar, author of *Light on Yoga,* which has become the Bible to the yoga world, says about the breath:

> The yogi's life is not measured by the number of his days but by the number of his breaths. Therefore, he follows the proper rhythmic patterns of slow deep breathing. These rhythmic patterns strengthen the respiratory system, soothe the nervous system and reduce craving. As desires and cravings diminish, the mind is set free and becomes a fit vehicle for concentration.[2]

We believe that Joseph Pilates understood this concept very well.

chapter 6

Mommy's Little Powerhouse
How to Share Pilates with Your Baby

*"I just can't get over how much babies cry.
I really had no idea what I was getting into. To tell you the truth,
I thought it would be more like getting a cat."*

———————

Anne Lamott,
Operating Instructions: A Journal of My Son's First Year,
Ballantine Books, 1994, p. 66

Your mat's down. Your water bottle is full. Your two blankets are propped up perfectly. Music is playing softly in the background. You're all ready to welcome your little workout partner. You get into position, place your baby on the mat and—lo and behold!—your baby bursts into tears. Now what?

A dose of flexibility, calm, and creativity is often all it takes to turn your baby into a cooperative partner. In this section, we will offer some general suggestions along with some more specific tricks to coax your baby to get with the program. The challenge is to adjust your workout to your baby's ever-changing state of mind, matching your own rhythm and tone to the shifts in your baby's moods. Your mission here is to create an atmosphere that is enticing to your baby while allowing yourself the optimal workout. Achieving this feat is an ongoing balancing act. You will save yourself a lot of unnecessary grief if you recognize from the outset that this is not something you can completely control. PeeWee Pilates is a far cry from running on a treadmill. With your baby in tow, you can never predict what will happen from moment to moment. On the bright side, every workout offers you and your baby a new adventure. Your baby's companionship ensures that the exercises will never get too routine or stale. In fact, the built-in flexibility invites you to be spontaneous and playful with your baby. Nothing is as reinforcing for both you and your baby as shared fun. You have license here to be as creative and light-hearted as you can while you interact with your baby. Feel free to sing, throw kisses, name body parts, or move to the cadence of a nursery rhyme, all while you're executing your Pilates movements. In other words, consider this simultaneously play time and work time, both for you and your baby. It's multitasking at its best!

Timing Is Everything

The first rule of thumb is to be attentive to your baby's moment-to-moment shifts in mood and needs. Babies can get cranky, colicky, hungry, wet, sleepy, distracted, or fussy according to their own time clock. PeeWee Pilates, of course, must take a backseat to your baby's own insistent demands. Timing is everything. Don't schedule your workout when your baby is hungry or just getting ready for a nap. (This may be a perfect time for you to work out on your own or catch up on some sleep yourself.) Most babies favor a period of time during the day when they are most alert and sociable; for some it is early morning, whereas for others it could be after their mid-afternoon nap. Those of you who are nursing may wish to feed your baby before you start working out so that you don't have to deal with the discomfort of engorged breasts. If you do need to stop and nurse or diaper your baby, you can resume your routine right afterward. Just be sure your baby has a moment to digest or you might end up with a face full of spit-up.

Some Days Are Better than Others

It is important to maintain a sense of humor and a willingness to improvise in your quest to reach greater fitness heights with a baby in tow. There will be days when your baby just can't get enough lifting or rolling around with you on the mat and could continue the exercises long after you've exhausted yourself. Then there are those days when she only wants to repeat a movement like "Rolling like a Ball" over and over again ad nauseam and nothing else will do. And sometimes, of course, you'll have the less pleasant experience of finding that nothing at all works to engage your baby. You could turn yourself upside down, make silly faces, massage your baby's limbs, and sing a full opera and still fail to persuade your baby to stop screaming.

Minimum Requirements

When your baby has had enough, you should at least try to plow through the "stomach series." In fact, we suggest that the stomach series become part of your daily habit, either solo or as a duet with your little one. In a matter of only five minutes, a frenzied mother can perform this group of five or six exercises that focus on the abdomen. Beyond the stomach series, depending upon your baby's frame of mind, you may have to mix and match your routine if your baby shows signs of protest. Over time, you will discover which exercises you and your baby prefer to do together and you may be able to prolong your workout simply by altering the sequence of the movements to keep your baby as content as possible. Such flexibility should help you keep your own frustration and anger at a minimum. Remember, too, that you only need to do ten or less repetitions of each movement; any more than this can threaten the integrity of your alignment. Besides, ten repetitions done with absolute concentration and alignment are far superior to a hundred sloppy crunches.

Dynamic Duo: Staying Engaged with Your Baby

Without uttering one single word, your baby is able to communicate her various desires, needs, and interests to you. As she smiles or frowns, gazes at you, or looks away, coos, frets, or giggles, she is "telling" you all about her shifting state of mind and "asking" you to respond to her. While you're working out, pay attention to what your baby is saying and honor her communications with a reply. Your baby wants nothing more than to engage in an ongoing communication dance with you. Recognize and reinforce these attempts to interact with you. As you reciprocate, try to calibrate your own responses to match her mood. If you sense that your baby is craving some high-intensity action, you may want to crank up the volume a bit, becoming a ham, moving more dramatically, making sillier sounds. Then, as you sense that your baby has had enough stimulation, slow it down a bit, and respect her need for quiet time or cooling off. Remember that babies strive for an optimal level of excitement and their moods can change as they try to strike this balance. By helping your baby tolerate and enjoy increasing amounts of stimulation and then helping her to calm herself afterward, you will teach her how to regulate her emotions on her own.

How do you know if your baby has had more than his share of stimulation at any one time? Look for the following signals: squirming, shutting eyes, turning his head away, evading your gaze, wrinkled brow, drowsiness, and of course crying.

"Help! I'm Gonna Have a Meltdown"

If your baby does start to fuss or cry during your workout, you may want to consider one of the following suggestions:

- Change positions. By just shifting the way you hold your baby, you're providing him with a new vestibular sensation and a new visual image to check out. These simple novelties may be enough to distract your baby. Try out different positions; some babies may be very particular and other babies more fickle about what they like and don't like.
- Adding a rocking motion can quiet your baby
- Stand up: Some babies may stop crying if you scoop them up and stand up. This could be a good time to do the "standing pliés."
- Offer exercises with more chest-to-chest contact, cuddling, or embracing. When you rest your baby's chest against your own, your baby can feel the soothing, familiar rhythm of your heartbeat.
- Shift your baby into an upright position. When you hold your baby's head upright, it can often help him settle down and focus. As Daniel Stern, psychiatrist and infant researcher, explained, "Putting a baby into the upright position is, for his nervous system, like switching gears in a car. He becomes quieted physically, but more alert mentally in the sense of being more open to the sights and sounds around him.[1]
- Shift your baby to "tummy time": Some babies, especially those with colic or gastroenterological distress, may feel more comfortable being placed on their stomachs. Interestingly, although colicky babies often prefer this position, mellower babies may not.[2]
- But if your baby fusses while in tummy-time position, you may try the following:
  1. Give a gentle push on his sacrum or lower back. This will help him arch his back.

2. Give reassuring strokings.

3. Place your baby on *your* chest instead, especially if he is a young infant, so that he experiences tummy time comforted by the touch of your chest.

- Try some of your baby's "favorite" movements. Some of the more popular ones are Rolling Like a Ball, Single Leg Kicks, PeeWee Teasers, Side Kicks, and the Tootsie Roll.

- Stop to feed your baby and then resume your workout.

- Give your baby a soothing massage. Just make sure that your touch is not too light or feathery. Tickling can distract or irritate your baby.

- Follow some of the suggestions on pages 79–81 to make your exercises more playful.

- Give special attention to your baby's highly sensitive body parts, such as your baby's face, palms, backbone, and soles of the feet.[3]

Safety First

Your baby's age and developmental pace are obviously going to have an effect on how you work out together. When your infant is very young, you will need to be mindful of her limited abilities, especially her immature muscular strength and her lack of neck and head control. Keeping your baby safe, it should go almost without saying, is of prime concern. You need to make sure that you hold your baby securely enough so that she does not flop back on her head or fall off your lap. Until your baby demonstrates adequate neck control, make sure that her head is not torqued forward or backward and her cervical spine is straight. Don't forget that your infant's head comprises a huge part of her body weight. A young infant doesn't yet know how to self-correct her position and work against gravity if her head is not positioned properly. The sensory input she needs to correct her position is not yet mature. If your baby is in a seated position, support her neck and back by firmly positioning your hands under her armpits and cupping them together at her neck.

Some additional words of caution:

- Avoid holding your baby's head below the rest of his body for more than a few moments; this position can cause blood to pool in your baby's head.
- Don't fling your baby around or use jerky motions as you move through the exercises. Your baby is not a rag doll. Try to move smoothly as you're shifting his position. Abrupt movements can be startling to some babies.
- Hold your baby firmly and try to handle him in a secure, confident manner.
- Don't try to force your baby to move beyond what he is able to do easily.
- Remember that babies like to be held close to their mother's body, preferably against their skin, so that they can smell her, feel her body heat, listen to her heart beat, and peer into her face. Most mothers also find that holding their babies closer to their center is more comfortable, especially for their posture. If you hold your baby too far away from your body, you may place unnecessary strain on your back, neck, and shoulders.[4]

The Changing Needs of Your Growing Baby

Over the course of your baby's first year of life, he evolves at an incredibly rapid rate from a seemingly helpless pooping machine into a more personable, chatty little person capable of deliberate movement, long periods of alertness, and full locomotion. The age of your baby will obviously shape the nature of your workouts together. While exercising with a younger baby, you might get the distinct impression that he is a passive passenger while you are working your butt off. As your baby becomes increasingly alert, physically active, and socially engaged, your workouts will naturally become a livelier, more dynamic partnership. The older baby may sometimes prefer to explore the area around you as you work out, entertaining himself in your close, comfortable presence, or he might become a more formidable playmate.

Newborn to Three Months Old

As a newborn, your baby starts out primarily in the fetal position; his movements are uncontrolled and jerky, he can only move his head from side to side, and he cannot support his head on his own. He can see only about eight to ten inches ahead of him, he has trouble tracking objects, and he sleeps most of the time. Don't be fooled, however, into thinking that your baby is a mindless blob. Remember that he can already recognize your voice, face, and scent and already has a reflex that encourages him to turn his head in the direction of a sound. At about two months, your baby will begin to delight you with his social smile, and between two and three months, he will start cooing. By about three months, your baby can begin to stretch and bend his arms and legs, his fingers have begun to uncurl, and he has started to bat at objects.

With a young baby, your interactions will be more gentle or low-key, as you and your baby begin to get to know each other through an exchange of eye contact, facial expressions, odor, touch, and sounds. Don't forget that you are performing an essential function as you hold him and move him about with you. As Stanley Greenspan stated, your function as a parent in the first months of your baby's life is basically to "help your baby look, listen, begin to move, and calm down."[5] Remember during your workouts to maintain frequent eye contact with your baby, talk to him about what you two are doing together, and respond to his shifting moods by adjusting your movements accordingly.

Three to Six Months Old

Your baby is now starting to become noticeably more attached to you and will increasingly try to engage you in progressively more elaborate "conversations" through smiling, cooing, and gestures. At four months, he will start chatting with you and will laugh when tickled, and by six months, his babbling will start to sound more as if he's really talking. During this span of time, your baby also develops increasing control over his upper body. By four months, he begins to show signs of neck and head control and enjoys being held in a sitting position (but can't yet support himself in this position). With increased muscle tone throughout his torso, at five months, your baby can roll back and forth from his stomach to his back and by six months may even be able to support himself while in a seated position, if only for a few wobbly moments. As you work out with a baby of this age, don't forget to offer lots of tummy time.

Playful ways to engage your younger infant:

- When your baby is on his back, play patty cake to gently open and close his arms.
- With your baby on his back, gently move his legs back and forth as if he is pedaling a bicycle. This movement promotes muscle development in his legs. Do not extend your baby's legs outward in a straddle any wider than his hips or shoulders. This forced extension can dislocate his hip joints. You can apply the same Pilates principles of alignment here; always work *within* your baby's frame.
- Play simple imitation games with your baby. Try sticking out your tongue or opening your mouth wide and see if your baby copies you.

As your baby grows, you can make your movements more complex; you might try moving your whole face around in a circle.[6] You may also try to imitate some of your baby's gestures and sounds. When he gurgles, mimic that sound. When he flares his fingers, repeat that gesture yourself. If your baby shows any signs of playing along with you in these imitation games, make sure to reward him handsomely with praise!

- Bring along a rattle.
- Name body parts: As you notice your baby discovering or reaching for a body part, name that part. You can also talk to him about what parts of the body you are using.
- Play peekaboo.
- Play sound games like "getting the engine started," making tongue trills, clicking, or clucking sounds.
- With your baby lying on his tummy, you might try to encourage pre-crawling by uncurling his hands and putting his hands down against the floor. If you press your baby's open palms down, you give your baby practice feeling the hard surface of the floor.

Six to Twelve Months Old

In the second half of your baby's first year, he will become much more interested in exploring the world around him and can't wait to get his hands on everything. As he gains control of his whole body and gains muscle strength, he is eager to practice his new motor skills and assert his newfound independence. Welcome to your nonstop moving baby! By about eight months, your baby is likely to sit on his own, crawl all about, and pick up objects with just his thumb and index finger. By ten months, your baby may be cruising and by twelve months may be walking or just on the verge of taking his first step. Along with his increasing autonomy, your baby's attachment to you is still paramount, and at about nine months, he develops stranger anxiety. Socially your baby will initiate play with you rather than waiting for you to get the ball rolling. By anywhere between nine and twelve months, your baby may enthrall you with his first word.

Playful ways to engage your older baby:

- Perform exercises in front of a mirror so your baby can watch both of your images together.
- The following exercises are a favorite of older babies: Rolling Like a Ball, Single Leg Kick, Standing Pliés, PeeWee Teasers, Side Kicks, and the Tootsie Roll. During the stomach series, you can add in baby presses where your baby is up in the air pressed away from you.
- Play peekaboo.
- Play more elaborate imitation games.
- Bring in toys. Your baby now loves to explore different objects.
- Engage in "name play," naming the objects, people, or activities that attract your baby's attention.

The key is to have fun together. If your baby does not seem to react to a game or a particular interaction with pleasure, it may mean that he is simply not developmentally ready to play. Don't feel that you have to impose it on him. Often, if you just wait a few days or weeks, your baby will have a complete change of heart.

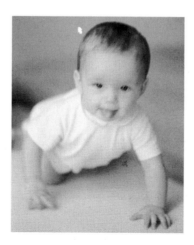

Part III

Getting to the Core
The Exercises

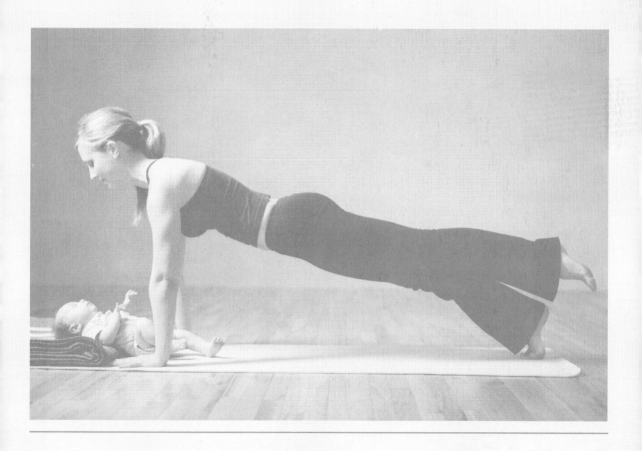

chapter 7

Pre PeeWee Pilates

PeeWee Pilates Exercises You Can Begin Right Away

Kegels

A Kegel—not to be confused with a kugel (a noodle casserole)—is the ideal exercise for strengthening your pelvic floor. Essentially what you do is contract your pelvic muscles as if you are trying to stop peeing midstream. "Unfortunately, the vast majority of women who are told to do Kegel's exercises are not instructed in how to do them properly," wrote Dr. Christiane Northrup, "and that's why so many women (and their doctors) don't think they work. When properly and consistently done, these exercises have been found to help up to 75% [of] women overcome their SUI (stress urinary incontinence) problems."[1] Dr. Northrup argued that all that Kegel work won't amount to much if you contract your abdominals, thighs, or buttocks at the same time that you're squeezing the vaginal area. The correct way to perform Kegels is to squeeze, for a count of three, those muscles that you use to stop the flow of urine. Take a momentary break, then squeeze these muscles once more. Try to increase the length that you hold the contraction

until you can hold each one for a full count of 10. Try to complete five sets
three times a day. (You may write us a thank you note later on behalf of your
sex life!) The beauty of the Kegels is that you can do them anywhere and no
one has to know what you're up to. Although it is commonly recommended
that you start Kegels immediately after giving birth, Dr. Russell, our consulting obstetrician, believes that it is more realistic to wait until about six
weeks after a vaginal delivery, by which time the inflammation around your
pelvic floor should subside and you will be better able to isolate your muscles. Even after this waiting period, it can be very difficult to discern
whether you are contracting the correct muscles. To check that you're performing the Kegels properly, it has been suggested that you place a finger
or two in your vagina while you squeeze your muscles.

Pre-Hundreds Breathing

Lie flat on your back with your knees bent and your feet flat on the floor.
Make sure that your entire spine is flat on the mat. Pull your navel deep in
toward your spine and try to "hide" your ribcage so that your ribs aren't
poking out. Place your arms at your sides, and push your palms flat against
the floor while lifting your fingers away from floor. This movement will engage your shoulder blades down your back and help relieve tension in your
shoulders. The entire length of your arms should be pressing back into the
floor so that your shoulders move back and down and the front of your
chest remains open. Don't hunch your shoulders! It may seem as if you're
not doing very much beyond holding this position using the floor as a resistance. While holding this position, focus on your breathing. (Some people choose to close their eyes to help them concentrate.) Inhale slowly and
evenly through your nose for a full five counts (one Mississippi, two Mississippi, etc.), and then exhale fully through your nose for another five counts
at the same slow speed. In other words, inhale 1-2-3-4-5, exhale 1-2-3-4-5.

Make it *one long continuous breath*. Do not hyperventilate. If this feels like too much, start with three counts in and three counts out until you can work your way up to five. Try to build up eventually to ten sets of inhaling and exhaling the full count for a total count of 100. This exercise is preparing your diaphragm (and your mind) for the deep and concentrated breathing that Pilates requires. It will also prepare you for the Hundreds, the exercise you'll start with when you are ready to begin PeeWee Pilates.

Pelvic Tilt

Follow the exercise above. Add on: As you inhale for a count of five, keeping your feet flat on the ground, pull your spine under and up, starting with your tailbone. Continue peeling your spine off the floor one vertebra at a time until you are midway up the spine (right where your bra strap is). Then as you exhale for five full counts, starting with the middle vertebra that is up roll down one vertebra at a time until your tailbone is flat on the floor again. Repeat 4 to 8 times.

Diastasis Rx

Lie flat on your back with your knees bent and your feet flat on the floor.

Pull your navel deep down toward your spine to maintain a flat back. *Don't arch.* Bring your hands to your rib cage. Push the sides of your abdominals in toward each other as if you're trying to close your rib cage into itself. Holding that position, inhale through your nose for three to five counts. As you exhale (again through your nose), lift your head up off the floor and bring your chin to your chest, looking at your belly button. Keep pulling your stomach muscles down tight while you are holding this forward position.

If you have a rubber Thera-Band or yoga strap, place it behind your back around your lower rib cage, and hold onto the ends in front of you. Grab each end of the strap with the opposite hand and give a light pull (it should feel as if it cinches your rib cage in—like a corset or a belt). As you bring your head forward, pull the strap a little tighter to encourage your abdominal wall to engage deeper and to gently close the gap where the separation occurred.

chapter 8

The PeeWee Pilates Exercises

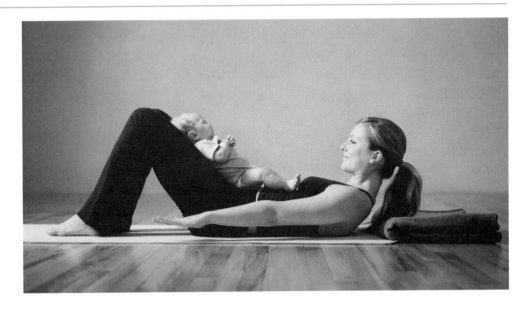

Mom's Placement: Place your folded blanket under your head. Lie flat on your back with your knees bent and your feet flat on the mat, hip width apart. (The width between your hips should be about two fists between your knees. Don't worry; no matter how fat you feel, your hips are not any wider apart than that!)

Baby's Placement: Cradle your baby on your thighs so that she is on her back leaning against your legs looking up at you.

Now What?

1. Lift your head forward until your chin is gently pressing on your chest. Make sure your neck is off the mat, gently rounding forward. You should be staring at your baby's belly button. Try to feel your neck stretching rather than straining. (Straining hurts; stretching should not.) If you need to, put your hands behind your neck and pull your head forward all the way off the floor.

2. Raise your arms up by your sides about two inches above your stomach. Extend your arms in one nice, straight line from the fingertips all the way up to the shoulders. Slide your shoulder blades down toward

your tailbone. This can be tricky to establish. It might help to imagine that you are pulling the tips of your wings together behind you.

Leave your head on the blanket instead of leaning it forward. Otherwise, follow the same arm pumping and breathing instructions, keeping your stomach muscles fully engaged.

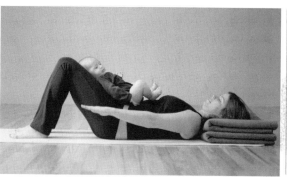

C - S E C T I O N   T I P

3. Keeping your head forward and your arms straight, now scoop out your stomach muscles, pulling them down to your spine. Here you might think of a bowl of soup resting inside the cavity of your belly. Deflate your rib cage.

4. Vigorously and repeatedly pump your arms straight up and down as if you are dribbling a small ball or you're trying to stay afloat in water. Keep your arms slightly above your stomach muscles and limit your range of motion to about three inches. Take five counts to inhale and five counts to exhale. Perform a total of ten sets (for a total of 100 pumps).

"C'mon," you quip, "there's no way my baby is scaling any major developmental heights right now while he's just lying there!" Wrong! While you're pumping away, your baby may be busy at work studying your face. Babies are prewired from birth to be strongly attracted to faces. As a one- or two-month-old, your baby is drawn to stark contrasts; to him, the darkness of your mouth, the light in your eyes, and the silhouette of your hairline can be as compelling as the *Mona Lisa* itself. After two months of age, your baby focuses more on the internal features of your face; he will be content to ponder for minutes at a time the unique angle of your nose or the lovely shape of your mouth. As he is examining your face, your baby is both developing his visual acuity and seeking your attention. Your older baby, in your secure presence, may now be more interested in looking elsewhere.

PeeWee Perspective

How Do You Know If You're Doing It Correctly?

Your entire spine should be pressed against the mat with no air pockets. If you feel any arching, you are not curling forward enough from the upper half of your body.

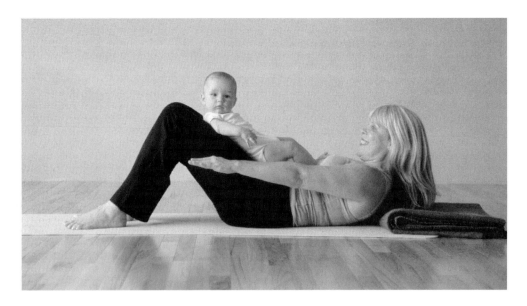

Mother's Little Helper: The Hundreds is the perfect place to start your Pilates workout. It is designed to warm up the body and calm down the mind. Your breath is key. But remember, ladies, this isn't Lamaze class! Your breath should be one long inhale and one long exhale through your nose. Even though you're pumping your arms, you're not pumping your breath. Don't exhaust yourself with spasmodic breathing. What new mother doesn't need to stop and take a deep breath to calm her nervous system? Besides, a calm mother makes for a calmer baby.

If you would foster a calm spirit, first regulate your breathing; for when that is under control, the heart will be at peace; but when breathing is spasmodic, then it will be troubled. Therefore, before attempting anything, regulate your breathing on which your temper will be softened, your spirit calmed.

—**Kariba Ekken, seventeenth-century mystic**[2]

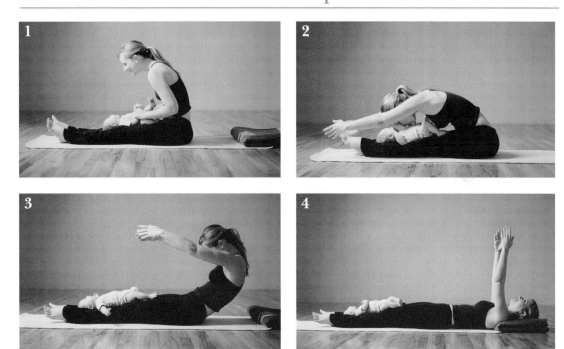

Mom's Placement: Sit up with your legs straight out in front of you in Pilates stance (heels together, toes apart).

Baby's Placement: Lay your young baby (under three months) flat on her back on your thighs, with her feet closest to you. If your baby shows neck control (usually at about three months and older), have your baby sit up. Hold onto your baby's hands or behind his neck if he needs extra support.

Now What?

1. Keeping your elbows slightly bent and squeezing your butt, pull your tummy in tight. Think of sliding your stomach up into your rib cage while you pull your navel back into your spine. Lower your chin onto your chest.

2. Slowly roll backward down your spine, one vertebra at a time, until you are flat on the mat. Rest your head on your blanket. Your older

baby should be sitting up at this point. A younger baby continues to
rest on your legs (see photo 4).

3. Now lift your chin forward toward your chest. Slowly roll up the spine,
curling forward, still pulling your powerhouse tight. Peel your spine

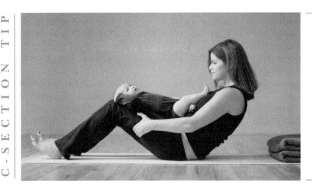

Bend your knees slightly and place
your hands behind your thighs to
hold on. Rest your baby on your
thighs, using your arms flanked on
both sides to create a secure hold for
him or her. Roll up in a straight line,
trying to keep from jerking your body
up or leaning from side to side.

off your mat, one vertebra at a time, until you are reaching all the way
forward toward your feet. As you stretch forward again, your baby will
gently roll back onto your legs. In other words, your baby rolls up and
down in opposition to your movements. If you have a younger baby,
she may prefer just resting on your thighs while you roll down and up.

4. Repeat to roll down.

For the younger baby, who remains on his back throughout this exercise, your alternating
appearance and disappearance over his face becomes a kind of peekaboo. Peekaboo offers a small baby a beginning opportunity to investigate how people or objects can exist
even when momentarily out of sight. Your baby very quickly learns to expect your face to
repeatedly reappear. Remarkable as it may seem, babies as young as two or three months
of age can recognize that there's a pattern to your crazy rolling behavior.

Older babies can become more active players in this exercise. By about five months, babies develop enough strength in their neck, shoulder, chest, and abdominal muscles so
that they're able to momentarily sit up. With your baby in a seated position and as you
hold onto his back or hands, your baby rolls down and up with you like a seesaw. Notice
how your older baby learns to anticipate the sequence. To add complexity to your "pattern" of movements, try making a silly face and sound every *other* time that you roll up.

PeeWee Perspective

How Do You Know If You're Doing It Correctly?

- Keep a "C curve" as you stretch. (You literally want to mold your spine into the letter *C* as your belly gets hollowed out.)
- As you roll down onto the mat, imagine you are rolling down into sand and you are trying to make an impression of your spine.
- This exercise can be quite challenging, but you've got the advantage of your baby acting as a weight to keep your lower body grounded.

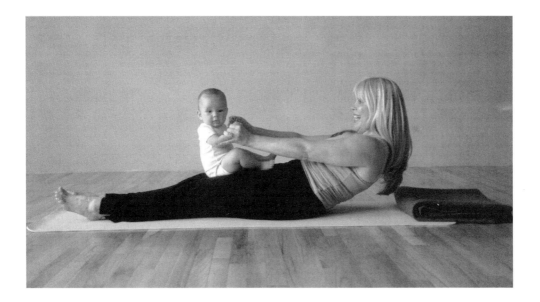

Mother's Little Helper: In the words of Joseph Pilates, "You are only as old as your spine." What he essentially meant is that the key to vitality lies in the flexibility and elongation of the spinal column. Look at your baby's wondrous agility. Think of his spine as your role model as you reach for maximum flexibility in your own spine. As we age, our backs become increasingly stiff and unforgiving. The best way to fight time is through rolling movements that open up the spine, one vertebra at a time, to prevent fusion. Pilates can help you regain flexibility and counteract the stiffening aging process.

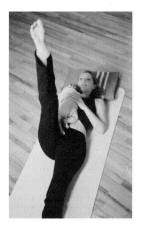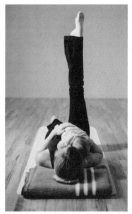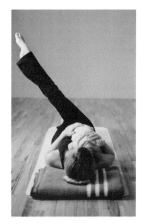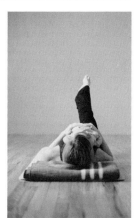

Mom's Placement: Lie flat on your back with a folded blanket under your head. Stretch your legs straight out ahead of you on the floor and turn your feet out in Pilates stance (heels together, toes apart).

Baby's Placement: Lie a younger baby on her tummy against your chest or stomach. Hold your baby with both hands around her head or waist, depending upon her need for neck support. If your baby is willing and able to sit up, have her sit on one leg (the nonworking one) as a weight. Keep her neck supported with your hands if she needs it.

Now What?

1. With one leg staying extended on the floor, bend the other leg in toward your chest and then lift it straight up into the air. Turn the top of your leg out from the hip so that you can see the inside edge of your foot facing you (rather than the top of the foot). This turnout from the hip will make sure that your inner thighs are fully engaged and working instead of relying on your quadriceps.

2. Draw small circles in the air with your leg by sweeping the extended leg across your body toward your opposite shoulder, then down toward the floor, and finally back up toward its starting point. Don't let this leg go beyond the frame of your shoulders. Start with a fairly small circle but feel free to widen it as you gain comfort and strength. Do

between five and ten circles with the right leg going counterclockwise first and then reverse the circle. Then change legs and do the same.

Modify by bending the leg on the floor and pushing that foot flat into the floor. Keep the circles very small, with the working leg and both hips very still.

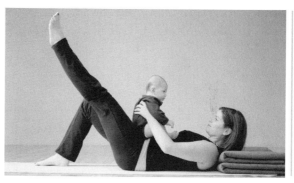

C - S E C T I O N   T I P

3. While you're circling each leg, pay attention to the rest of your body. It should be completely still and stable. Your navel should be pulled down to your spine, with your rib cage trying to sink into your body and both of your hips pressed against the floor. Your other leg, the one extended on the floor, should push against the floor, thereby helping to anchor

This position offers multisensory pleasures for a young baby. Your baby gets to smell your neck (a baby's favorite smelling spot, according to our pediatrician consultant Dr. Geary), feel your heart beating against his chest, see into your eyes, and maybe even hear your breathing.

In an amazingly short amount of time, your baby develops from this sweet, contemplative perceiver and processor of his environment to a performer in his own right. Babies are able to imitate others practically from birth, and as they get older, they learn to use others as a kind of social mirror to teach them novel ways of doing things. On the following page, Charly, at eight and a half months old, appears to be trying to copy her mother; she explores her own foot while her mother's foot circles overhead. Give her a few months and she may put her leg up in the air, too! Remember that babies learn a to just from watching what they see other people do. By about eight months of age, b even develop an ability to recall something that they've seen before withou prompted by a reencounter with it.[3] So be mindful of what you do!

PeeWee Perspective

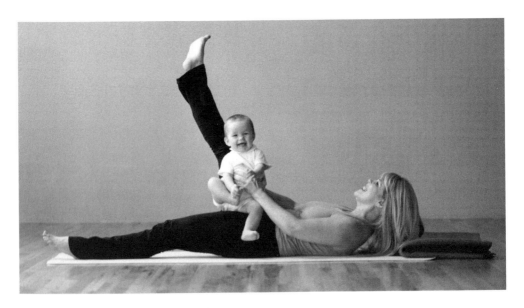

your body. Imagine you are lying down in an earthquake and trying to use your body weight against the shaking floor to stay still. Don't give in!

How Do You Know If You're Doing It Correctly?

- You should feel the inner thigh tightening from the turnout in the hip. Notice the operable word here: *turnout!* We can't stress that enough for this one. The circle should stay within the frame of your

Mother's Little Helper: Notice here that although Charly may be imitating her mama, they are not directly interacting. Don't feel as if you have to interact nonstop with your baby. Especially in an exercise like this, where you have to concentrate on keeping so much of your entire body engaged and still, it's OK to focus primarily on your own body ⏤oments. In fact, researchers have found that your baby is more likely to feel ⏤ if you do *not* lavish her with *absolute, unwavering,* hypervigilant at- respond to every single little motion, gesture, or sound that ⏤ unwittingly undermine their baby's developing capacity to ⏤s as well as their baby's desire to pursue independent activity. ⏤by enjoy her own explorations in your safe proximity while you ⏤our core.[4]

shoulders. Do not take the circle wider than the shoulder on the same side as the working leg. Don't let the hip on the side of the working leg leave the floor; otherwise, you will have crossed your leg too far over your body and destabilized the pelvic floor.

- This exercise is about challenging your powerhouse by trying to keep the body stabilized while you are forming the leg circles. Therefore it is important not to flail your lifted leg. Keep your movements contained.

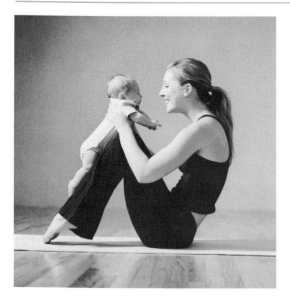 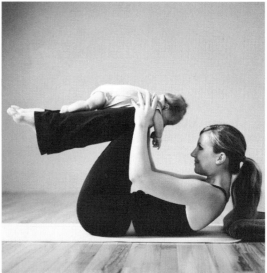

Mom's Placement: Sit up with your knees bent and pulled in close enough to you so that you can grab your ankles.

Baby's Placement: Rest your baby against your calves facing you so that he or she can peek out over your knees and look at you. Hold your baby securely under his or her arms.

Now What?

1. Lift your heels gently off the floor and balance on your toes or, if you can, with your toes in the air. Try to trust your balance. Pull your stom-

---

The rolling in this exercise provides your baby with lots of vestibular stimulation. When
~our baby about, you shift the fluid in her inner ear. This, in turn, triggers the
~nd a sensory message to her brain and spinal cord that her body
member (see page 52) that it is your vestibular system that
d and body posture, to successfully move parts of your body,
maintain balance. By stimulating your baby's vestibular sense,
our baby's visual attentiveness to the world around him and ac-
of his reflexes and his motor skills.[5]

PeeWee Perspective

ach in tight toward your back, imagining you have on a supertight pair of jeans and you don't want to bust out of them. Try to release your neck forward, leaning your chin on your chest.

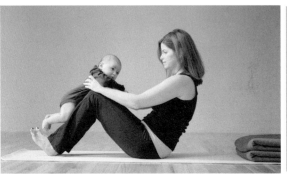

Keep your heels flexed on the floor and only roll down about halfway; then come right back up.

2. Roll back softly onto your spine. Roll only until you feel the lower half of your shoulder blades touch the mat. Do not roll onto your neck!
3. Pull your tummy in tight and roll immediately back up.

How Do You Know If You're Doing It Correctly?
- You should not use any momentum. Your legs should remain still.
- Be careful not to fall into a dead weight as you are rolling backward. Try to aim the crown of your head forward to maintain a rounded spine.
- Your baby will help you by keeping you from kicking your legs to roll back up.

Mother's Little Helper: During the last few months of your pregnancy, your lumbar spine most likely began to arch to accommodate the growing weight of your baby. The result of this strain can be tightened muscles and discomfort in the lower back area. (This is sometimes referred to as lordosis.) Unfortunately, throughout your pregnancy, you had very little opportunity to open up your lower back with deep forward bending because your baby was in the way. Not anymore. Rolling like a ball is one of the quickest ways to regain flexibility in the lumbar spine and to soothe your lower back. Having your baby on your legs actually helps you open up your back even more, giving you an even more pleasurable stretch. This exercise deserves a gold star.

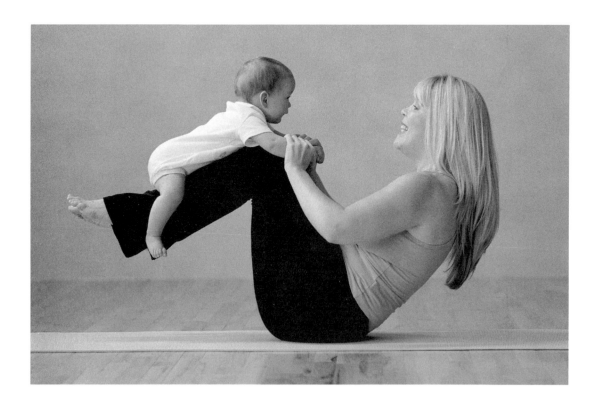

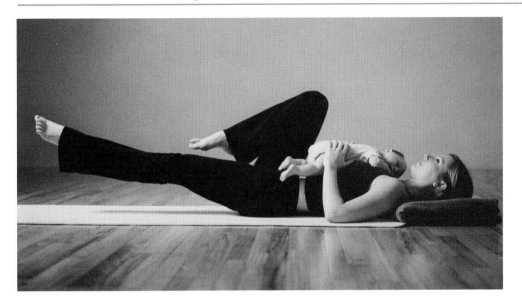

(#1 of the Stomach Series)

Mom's Placement: Lie flat on your back with your legs straight in front of you.

Baby's Placement: Hold your baby on your chest or in the air as if she is flying above you. Think of your baby as a weight that pushes your arms down and into your shoulder sockets. Don't let your shoulders lift up toward your ears.

Now What?

1. Bring your chin forward onto your chest. Bend the right knee into the chest as the left leg extends straight forward about six inches off the floor.

2. Alternating between legs, bend each knee into your chest and then extend your leg outward at an angle as close to the floor as you can, while keeping your back flat on the mat.

3. Inhale as you bend the right knee, and exhale as you bend the left. Complete ten sets on each leg.

How Do You Know If You're Doing It Correctly?

- Keep the feet long and relaxed. Try not to point or flex your feet, to ensure that your entire leg, all the way up to your hip, is working.

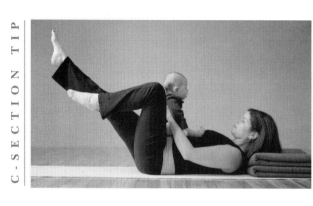

Keep your baby on your tummy. When you extend each leg, keep your leg lifted at a forty-five-degree angle or higher. This will help protect against strain on your incision.

- If your arms get too tired from holding your baby, lay her down on your tummy while you complete the exercises. The weight of your baby will remind you to keep your back flat against the mat.
- Rest your neck if it feels tired or strained, but try to keep it up for as long as possible. With just a little practice, you will notice much improved neck strength.

For the first four of these exercises, the younger baby remains in the prone position. This is an important prelude to official tummy time. Although he is not actively engaged on the floor, he can begin to practice pushing off your chest with his hands and lifting his head up, turning it from side to side.

If you have an older baby who has developed neck control and you are ready for an extra challenge, try pressing your baby up into the air as if he's flying, and hold him as long as you can. You can also use your baby as a weight to press up and down for a few repetitions. Many older babies *adore* being suspended above you and don't want to come down, even when your arms tire! In addition to offering a whole new view of you and the world around you, this postural and visual novelty gives your baby another excellent "vestibular" workout.

PeeWee Perspective

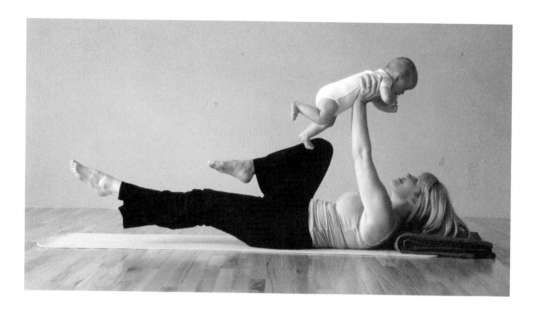

Mother's Little Helper: You have now entered the famous Pilates stomach series! This is a series of five exercises that Joseph Pilates designed for his students to do *every day* in this particular, fixed order. It is choreographed so that each exercise flows right into the next one with minimal extraneous movement during each transition. Think of it as your mini-Pilates workout on those days when you can't get to anything else. The stomach series works every single muscle of the powerhouse. If you just do these five exercises on a daily basis, with or without your baby, and get to nothing else, you will still see significant results in your midsection.

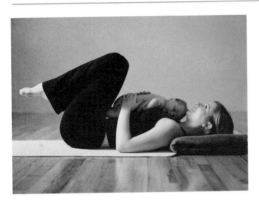 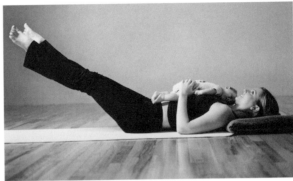

(# 2 of the Stomach Series)

Mom's Placement: Lie flat on your back with your legs stretched out in front of you on the floor and your feet turned out in Pilates stance (heels together, toes apart).

Baby's Placement: Place a younger baby on her tummy against your chest. An older baby can sit on your stomach facing you. Hold your baby securely and support her neck if needed. Try to keep your elbows pulling down tightly in toward your body. This keeps your shoulders down and engages the triceps (or the chicken wings).

Now What?

1. Bring your head forward off the blanket and try to reach your chin down to touch your chest. Press your navel down toward your spine and maintain a flat back. Hold your rib cage down as if you were tied into a corset.
2. Bend both knees simultaneously into your body.
3. As you inhale, extend both legs slowly outward until your legs are straight. Keep the extension fairly high in the air.
4. As you exhale, bend your knees back into your chest.
5. Repeat five to ten times.

How Do You Know If You're Doing It Correctly?

- You shouldn't feel any pain or arching in your lower back. If you do, you are probably extending the legs too low. Arching your lower back is a definite sign that your powerhouse is not fully engaged. Remember

Place your second folded blanket under your pelvis so that your lower back and hips are raised up on a slight angle. This will help to avoid any strain on your back or your incision that could result from any arching of the spine. Be sure to extend your legs *up* at a higher angle instead of forward, to avoid compromising the incision.

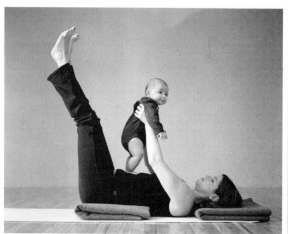

C - S E C T I O N   T I P

On the next page, notice the contentment that Charly, now almost nine months old, exudes during the workouts; she assumes this is *her* playtime. Because she has been participating in these workouts since she was about eight weeks old, she has learned to anticipate a particular flow to the routine. Routines can provide babies with an important sense of security, predictability, and order as well as offer a kind of "memory lesson."[6] However, it is important to make sure that the routine does not become too "old hat." Babies love novelty and are surprisingly good at recognizing when they've already seen some trick or heard some sound before. A preference for novelty encourages babies to seek out new stimulation that will in turn promote the development of new synaptic growth in the brain.[7] Try to keep things exciting by making subtle changes in the routine: Bring in new objects, change your background music, alter the rhythm of your movements, or try out new games (see pp. 75–81 for suggestions). You may also consider changing the location of the workout from time to time, such as from your bedroom to your living room (assuming you have the luxury to do so).

PeeWee Perspective

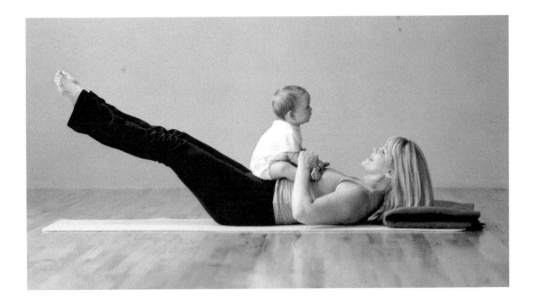

that you may have gotten all too comfortable arching your back throughout your pregnancy. It's time to start breaking that habit!

• Move as if you are underwater. Slowly, gracefully as if you're doing a beautiful backstroke. As you get stronger with time, challenge yourself to extend your legs lower and lower toward the floor.

Mother's Little Helper: While babies may enjoy relying on a routine, many new mothers do not exactly relish the prospect of sticking to a daily exercise regimen. However, a consistent workout doesn't have to entail a brutal hour of strenuous exercise every single day. In fact, just ten minutes of exercise has been shown to perk up your mood, decrease your fatigue, and instill a sense of vigor. After twenty minutes of exercise, increased mental clarity has also been demonstrated.[8] The stomach series is an ideal choice for a quick workout when you have little time or energy, and we recommend that you make it a non-negotiable daily routine, with or without your baby. Since there's no rolling on the spinal column, the stomach series can be done anywhere you like, provided you have a flat surface available. You may even find afterward that you now have enough energy to extend your workout by another ten or twenty minutes.

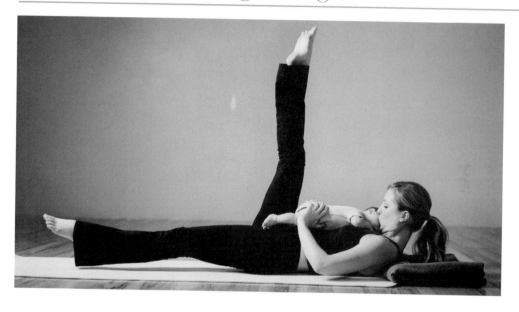

(#3 of the Stomach Series)

Mom's Placement: Lie flat on your back with your legs straight on the floor in Pilates stance.

Baby's Placement: Place a younger baby on her tummy against your chest. An older baby can sit on your stomach facing you. Hold your baby securely and support her neck if needed. Keep your elbows pulling down tightly in toward your body.

Now What?

1. Bring your head forward off the blanket and reach your chin down, trying to touch it to your chest. Press your navel and your rib cage down toward your spine, and maintain a flat back throughout this exercise.

2. Kick your right leg straight up in the air for two counts. Think of kicking up on the first count and then pulling it up slightly higher from there for the second count.

3. Switch the legs like scissors and do the same on the left side.

4. The lower leg should extend at least three to five inches off of the floor.

5. Inhale as the right leg kicks up. Exhale as the left leg kicks up.

6. Do five to ten sets.

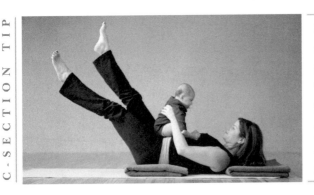

Place your second folded blanket under your pelvis to raise your hips slightly higher than your lower back. This will help keep you from arching in the low back as well as help to protect your incision from strain. Avoid taking the leg lower than forty-five degrees. If you feel any pain, *stop*.

How Do You Know If You're Doing It Correctly?

- The legs should stay long and straight from the hips to the feet. Try not to bend the knees or ankles. It will only make your legs feel heavy and harder to lift. Kick like a Rockette, not a football player!

- Move gracefully and gently, as if you're underwater. Avoid forceful movements.

When your baby is lying on her tummy in this face-to-face position (as on the previous page), the two of you have the perfect opportunity to enjoy an intimate moment together playing a game of imitation. If your baby is under three months of age, stick out your tongue, protrude your lips, or shake your head and see if your little monkey imitates you. (Babies can start doing this right from birth!)[9] If your baby is a little older, try to make your facial gestures more complicated. By six months of age, your baby may be able to re-member your expression and mirror it back to you a full day later.[10] We also encourage you to play with your baby's adorable sounds. Babies love to have their own vocalizations repeated by you and to receive useful feedback about how to make syllables and other sounds from your more precise imitations.

PeeWee Perspective

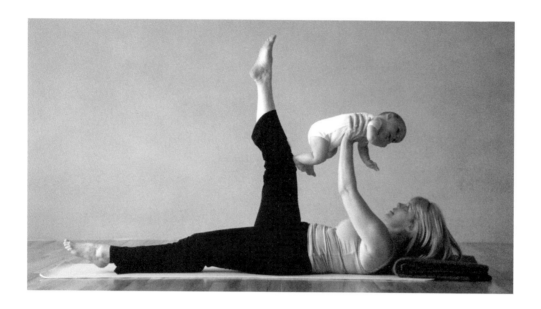

Mother's Little Helper: Many new moms are blown away by the intensity of their joyous, adoring, almost uncontrollable love for their new babies. As you commune with your baby, you may find, in fact, that you can become so absorbed in the momentary passion together that you lose a sense of time passing. Daphne de Marneffe, a clinical psychologist and author of *Maternal Desire*, explains: "The nowness of interacting with a child, or the absorption of looking into her face, can release us momentarily from our usual sense of time" and give us a "fleeting sense of eternity or boundarylessness."[11]

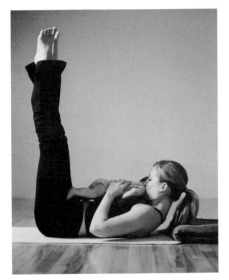 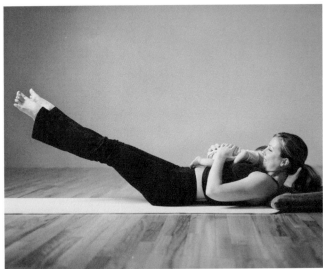

(#4 of the Stomach Series)

Mom's Placement: Lie flat on your back with your head on the folded blanket and your legs at a ninety-degree angle straight up in the air in Pilates stance. Keep the legs long and straight.

Baby's Placement: Place a younger baby on his tummy against your chest. An older baby can sit on your stomach facing you. Hold your baby securely and support his neck if needed. Keep your elbows pulling down tightly in toward your body.

Now What?

1. Keep your legs turned out and squeeze your inner thighs together as tightly as you can. (Pretend you've got the winning lottery ticket in there!) It doesn't hurt to squeeze your buttocks on this one as well.

2. Pull your navel to your spine and pull your spine down into the mat.

3. Bend your knees into your chest and then straighten your legs up into the air.

4. Lift your head forward off the blanket and press your chin onto your chest.

Skip this until your incision is well healed. When you are ready to begin, place your second folded blanket under your pelvis so that your lower back and hips are raised up on a slight angle. This will help you to avoid strain on your back or on your incision that could result from any arching of the spine. Be safe! Only lower your legs a few inches, and then, instead of lifting them straight up, bend your knees back into your chest. Take it easy!

5. As you inhale, slowly lower your legs down toward the floor. Keep your lower back strongly pressed against the mat.
6. As you exhale, slowly lift your legs back up to the ninety-degree angle.
7. Repeat up to ten times.

Because this especially challenging exercise requires so much concentration and effort, it is unlikely that you will remain the cheerful, attentive mom to your baby for these few moments that you're exerting yourself. Your loving, smiley face may suddenly tighten and you may momentarily turn away from your baby as you focus on your form. Don't expect this temporary change in your face and your affect to escape the notice of your exquisitely sensitive baby. Infants are surprisingly astute observers of adult social signals, particularly changes in your eye gaze, and shifts in your mood.[12] Babies as young as two or three months old can distinguish different emotions and come to expect their parent to interact with them in a distinctive style. Research has shown that if you suddenly change from happily interacting with an infant (even a baby as young as three months old) to putting on a "still face"—that is, a flat, blank expression—your baby is likely to react to this short-term "loss" of you. He may appeal to you to "come back to life" by moving his arms and legs, vocalizing, or exhibiting some other attention-seeking behavior.[13] However, in this exercise, your baby may be so puzzled by the contorted look on your face as you move your legs up and down that even he will not know what to make of you.

PeeWee Perspective

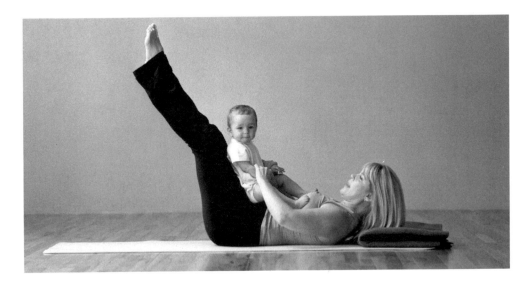

How Do You Know If You're Doing It Correctly?

- Start slowly with this one. In order to protect your lower back from strain, only take your legs as low as you comfortably can while maintaining a flat back. When you first attempt this exercise, lower your legs just a few inches and then slowly bring them back up. As you gain

Mother's Little Helper: Becoming a new mother is a lot like this exercise; it requires you to locate and activate strength, flexibility, and endurance in your core that you may never have known you could possibly possess. We believe, in fact, that discovering these buried reservoirs within you can be one of the most surprisingly satisfying treasures of motherhood. Despite being worn down from sleep deprivation, crying spells, and endless dirty diapers, most of the time (although, we all have our moments!) mothers can continue to summon from some unknown recesses of their brain nurturance, empathy, reasonably good judgment, and the juggling skills of a circus performer. According to journalist Katherine Ellison in her new book, *The Mommy Brain*,[14] this is no accident. She argues that the hormonal changes of motherhood, in combination with the powerful sensory experiences and emotional and physical responsibilities of being a mother, actually create a powerful transformation of a mother's brain. Drawing on several recent scientific studies, Ellison makes a convincing argument that motherhood actually improves your resilience, your emotional intelligence, your capacity to nurture, your level of efficiency, and more!

strength, you can make it more challenging by taking them lower. It may not look too impressive at first, but if you work slowly with good form, you will build strength without wrenching your back!

- Proper breathing is a lifesaver here. Inhale as you lower your legs; exhale as you lift. Breathe deeply through your nose without holding your breath. Let the movement follow the breath to avoid building tension in your body. Try to keep your movements slow and graceful, not forced or jerky.

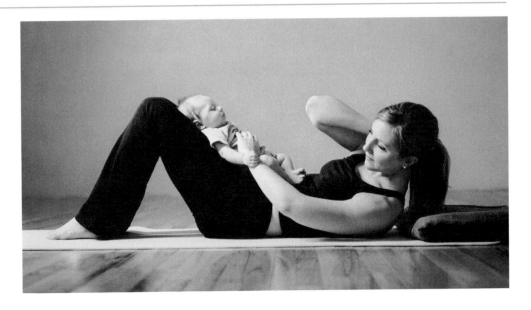

(#5 of the Stomach Series)

Mom's Placement: Lie flat on your back with your head on the blanket. Bend your knees and press your feet flat on the floor. Separate your feet and knees slightly (about a fist-width apart). Keep your feet a good distance away from your bottom.

Baby's Placement: Your baby should be sitting against your thighs, facing you, with her feet resting on your tummy and her head resting against your knees.

Another Option: Place your baby's tummy against your thighs, so she is facing away from you. She can rest her armpits over your knees. This is a good choice if your baby is a little cranky or colicky. Take a minute to give a little massage or pat her bottom gently to calm her.

Now What?

1. As you inhale, place your left hand against your baby's tummy (or back) and your right hand behind your neck.

2. As you exhale, keep your left hand on your baby; bring your head forward as you twist your torso over to the left.

3. Be sure to bring your right shoulder forward and off the mat as you reach your elbow across toward your left knee.

4. Inhale as you release back down to the starting position.

5. Repeat up to ten times, and then do the same on the other side.

No modifications here. We recommend that you wait until you are four or five months post-delivery before doing any twisting movements. Just be sure you are able to do this exercise without any pain or strain to your incision. Take it slow, and begin with a very small range on the twist for just a few reps. Stop if you feel any discomfort.

C-SECTION TIP

How Do You Know If You're Doing It Correctly?

- If you bend your knees too tightly, you won't be able to move well, and your baby will not have a good angle to lean against you.
- Keep your feet strongly pressed against the floor and your stomach pulled in tightly. When you twist, try to deflate your rib cage and try to

Don't forget to stop between exercises and reward your baby with a little massage. (See p. 47 to remind yourself of the extraordinary benefits of infant massage.) Massage your baby's body using your fingertips and the palms of your hands, making sure that your touch is not too light or tickling. Your baby's arms, legs, abdomen, chest, back, and even ears and face are all great places to rub, knead, or stroke. If you are in a warm enough room, you may want to take off some of your baby's clothing, allowing for skin-to-skin contact. You may even want to use some baby lotion or oil to eliminate annoying friction on your baby, but make sure to keep the lotion away from your baby's face.[15]

PeeWee Perspective

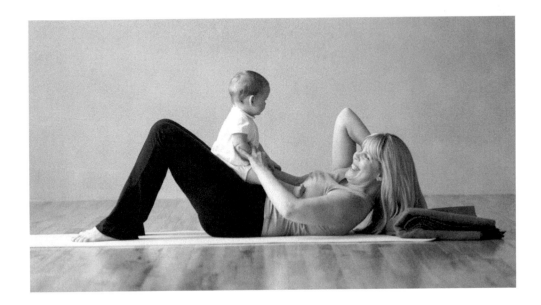

reach the lowest rib on your right side all the way over toward the left side of the room. The deeper you twist, the better the exercise works!

• The breathing may seem a little awkward at first. As a rule, you exhale into a twist. This squeezes more air out of your lungs and creates more space for a deeper twist and more effective use of the powerhouse.

Mother's Little Helper: While you're working those abs, let's look at that other major change in your abdominal region, namely your skin. Your belly may be saggy from the stretching it required to accommodate your uterus, you might have a darkened line of pigment, and to top it off, the stretch marks that seemed light and less noticeable while you were carrying your baby are now darker with a red tint and about as subtle as a Christmas tree! Don't worry, these marks usually fade with time. Your skin can begin healing from the inside out. One thing you can do to speed this process is to stay hydrated. Try to drink eight to ten glasses of water a day at a minimum. (Large amounts of water may also help with other postpartum ailments, such as edema, constipation, insomnia, irritability, and even carpal tunnel syndrome.)[16]

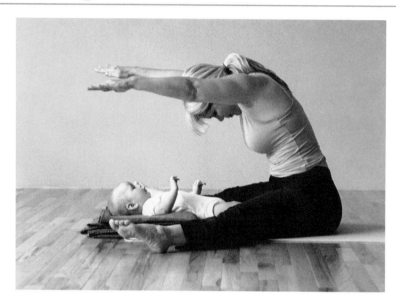

Mom's Placement: Sit up straight with your legs extended out in front of you. Open your legs so that the distance between them is as wide as your mat. If you find yourself slouching or cannot sit up with a very straight lower back, fold your blanket a few times and sit on the forward edge of it. This will keep your hips slightly higher than your legs so that you can pull up straight out of the lower back and hips.

Baby's Placement: Place your baby flat on his back facing you on a folded blanket between your legs. (Use a second blanket or a baby blanket if you are sitting on the folded one.)

Now What?

1. Extend your arms forward from your shoulders to your fingertips. Sit up as tall as you can and keep the shoulder blades pulling down toward your tailbone. Picture a zombie or Frankenstein's monster.

2. As you inhale, squeeze the muscles of your pelvic floor and buttocks. Try to sit on top of those muscles as if you're sitting on a bed of nails. Then pull your stomach in tight and try to lift your waist up off your hips. Continue with this growing feeling by squeezing your ribs toward

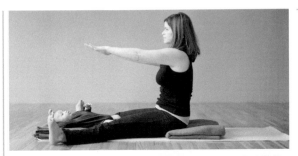

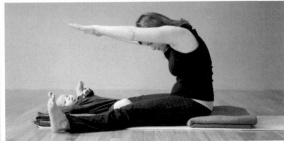

Sit on top of the folded blanket. When you first attempt this, just master the powerhouse engagement by following Step 2 above and then releasing. Add on the rest when you feel more comfortable. Work on mastering the breathing. Keep the forward bend modest, and really focus on tightening your abdominal wall back into your spine. The feeling of engagement may be hard to access in the beginning. Stick with it, and you'll feel it working with some time and patience.

each other and finally lifting your chest up toward your chin. Then lower your chin against your collarbone. Once you have all these muscles engaged, you will have your full powerhouse engaged. Yes, it's a lot of effort, but it's worth it!

3. As you exhale, pull your navel and rib cage further back into your spine, and hollow out the front of your torso. Keeping the full powerhouse engaged, stretch forward and down toward your baby by curl-

---

While lying on his back in front of you, your younger baby may be focused on his own exercise goals: exploring his own body, figuring out what it can do, and gaining control over his movements. Your baby's exercise program includes kicking his feet, grabbing his knees, turning his head, bringing his hands to his mouth, and waving them above his face. As random and repetitive as these movements may seem, they are really important attempts at both self-exploration and "practicing" behaviors that will prepare him to make more coordinated movements as he develops. Your baby figures out early on where his body begins and ends[17] and starts to discover that he is a separate physical being from you.[18] As he initiates his own movements, he also learns that, all by himself, he can *cause* things to happen by moving his little body.

PeeWee Perspective

ing in toward yourself. Think of reaching your nose into your belly button and the crown of your head toward your baby's tummy.

4. Your arms and hands should reach above your feet, and your head will drop between them. You should feel a deep stretch from the top of your neck all the way down your spinal column to your tailbone.

5. Now inhale again. Continue squeezing as you slowly unroll your spine, stacking up one vertebra at a time until you are back to the zombielike posture.

6. Finally, exhale as you relax and release all the squeezing and tightening of the powerhouse.

7. Repeat three to five times.

How Do You Know If You're Doing It Correctly?

When performing this exercise, imagine you are curling into yourself like a snail coiling into its shell. From the top of your spine to your tailbone, the profile of your body should resemble the letter *C*.

The most important thing here is to use your breath properly. This is a cleansing exercise for the lungs in addition to a stretch for the spine. Keep your mouth closed; instead, inhale and exhale to capacity through your nose. You should exhale so deeply that you feel you simply cannot push any more air out, as if you were a deflated balloon. This is how you get rid of the stale air in the lungs as well as increase your lung capacity. Exhaust your breath. You may even feel a little buzz after a few repetitions!

Mother's Little Helper: Although we don't mean to suggest that your baby is a pain in the neck, going about the business of caring for an infant may leave many mothers with tension and tightness in their necks, shoulders, and upper backs. As you lean over to breastfeed, lug your baby around with all his paraphernalia, and bend over strollers and cribs, you all too easily can strain your neck. Also, when tired or stressed, some people carry that tension around in the neck and shoulders. It can even migrate up to the head and turn into a terrible tension headache. Consider this exercise a relieving stretch to open the back of the neck and alleviate some discomfort.

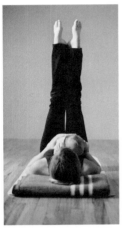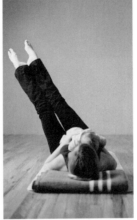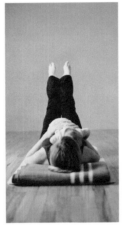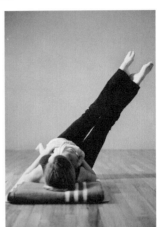

Mom's Placement: Lie flat on your back with your legs straight up in the air at a ninety-degree angle in Pilates stance. Leave your head down on your blanket for the entire exercise. Give your neck a welcome rest!

Baby's Placement: Place a younger baby on her tummy against your chest. An older baby can sit on your stomach facing you. Hold your baby securely and support her neck if needed. Keep your elbows pulling down tightly in toward your body.

Now What?

1. With your legs tightly together up in the air, squeeze your inner thighs and bottom, as well as your pelvic floor muscles.

2. Pull your navel to your spine, deflate your rib cage, and flatten your spine down to the mat.

3. Moving your legs as one unit, you will draw a small circle with your feet. Keep your legs nice and long from the hips to the feet. Try not to bend your knees or ankles. The length will help your legs feel lighter in the air and will discourage bulkiness in your leg muscles.

4. As you inhale, reach your legs a few inches over toward the right side of the room and start to circle them slowly down a few inches toward the floor.

5. As you exhale, continue the circle up and over to the left side of the room. The full circle should finish with your legs dead center at the top (back where they started out).

Don't try this modification until your incision is healed. When you are ready, place your second folded blanket under your pelvis to raise your hips slightly higher than your lower back. This will help keep you from arching your lower back.

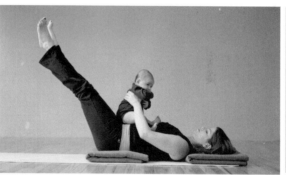

C - S E C T I O N   T I P

6. Now reverse the direction of the circle (breathing in as you circle toward the left and exhaling as you come up to the right).
7. Repeat for five or ten sets.

How Do You Know If You're Doing It Correctly?
- Visualize your legs as a mermaid tail. Your fins will stay open because you are holding the turnout from the inner thighs down to the feet. Now swing your tail around slowly to draw the circle and stabilize your entire torso throughout the exercise.

As your younger baby rests on your chest, notice how he positions himself. Each baby derives a sense of comfort and security in his own fashion. It is important to stay attuned to and respectful of your baby's own personal preferences. As pediatrician and psychiatrist Stanley Greenspan has observed, "Some babies curl up like kittens as you hold them against your chest; others flail their limbs or seem stiff-legged and tense when held in that position."[19] You may need to find out through trial and error which position is most relaxing to your baby. If he fusses while lying on you, see if he wants to sit up with your support.

PeeWee Perspective

- Be sure that you don't reach too far over or down. Your back should remain flat and your tailbone and hips should be glued to the mat. If the back of your left hip pulls away from the floor as you are circling the legs to the right, then you are reaching too far over. The circumference of the circle that your feet draw should be about the size of a basketball. As you get stronger, you can start to make the circle bigger. Just don't lose the integrity of your powerhouse!
- Don't let the name fool you. You draw one clear circle with your legs, not a figure-eight shape.

Mother's Little Helper: Your older baby can literally be your little helper on this one. By sitting on your belly, she essentially becomes your personal trainer, ensuring that you will keep your back flat. Her weight will help stabilize your powerhouse so you don't throw your hips around while your legs are circling.

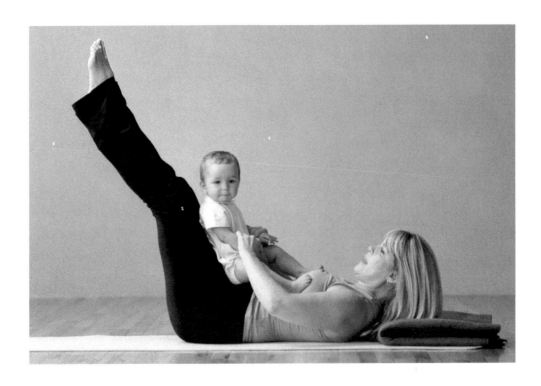

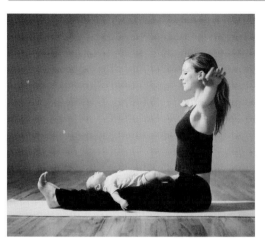
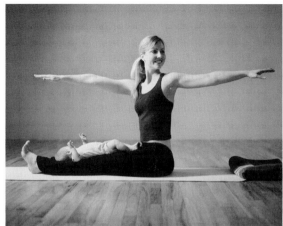

Mom's Placement: Sit with your legs extended straight in front of you close together. Legs should be *parallel* and with flexed feet (no Pilates stance this time). If you find yourself slouching or cannot sit up with a straight lower back, fold your blanket a few times and sit on the forward edge of it.

Baby's Placement: Place your baby on your thighs flat on her back facing you.

Now What?

1. Reach your arms straight out to the sides of the room. Imagine you have a broomstick that starts from one hand and runs across the top of your shoulders to the other hand. Keep your chest open and lifted.

2. Now imagine a second stick running the length of your spine from the tailbone all the way up to the top of your head. Keep your spinal column long and straight. Pull your rib cage in tight. Draw the shoulder blades down toward the tailbone. Try to lift the waist up off the hips and pull the ribs up off the waist. You should feel as if you have grown six inches.

3. As you inhale, sit on that bed of nails again! Flex your feet and squeeze the muscles of your hips, buttocks, and pelvic floor. Float on top of your buttock muscles.

4. As you exhale, twist to the right like a helicopter for two counts looking over your right shoulder. The first count will initiate the twist. The
second count will take the twist even deeper as you lift higher out of
your waist, reaching farther out of your fingertips and squeezing your
rib cage tighter into itself.

We recommend that you skip this one for now. Wait until your incision is fully
healed and then wait a little more! This is a deep twist that could compromise your
stitches and your newly healed incision or scar. Save this one for when you don't feel
the need to use the other C-section modifications.

5. Inhale as you come back to center and prepare to twist to the left, now
looking over your left shoulder.
6. Repeat sequence for three to five sets.

As your baby lies on your legs, your arms swinging above become a human mobile for her
to visually track. As you're twisting to and fro, this is a great opportunity to rhythmically
pair your movements with a joyful greeting. As you face forward, say, "Hello" to your baby,
and as you twist away, say, "Good-bye," and wave your hand. Remember that employing a
baby's multiple senses in unison presents optimal stimulation for her brain development.[20] Here you're combining the visual stimuli of your arms with your smiling face and
the sound of your exhaling breaths or your voice. Before five months of age, when your
baby has not yet mastered the ability to grasp objects, "his world is still confined to, designed for, and geared to interact with the 'sound and light show' that is his parent's vocal
and gestural behavior."[21] See if your baby responds to your "sound and light show" with
her own dramatic flourishes; she may chime in with her own sounds or even wave back.

PeeWee Perspective

How Do You Know If You're Doing It Correctly?

- Be sure to twist from your waist and not your hips! Your hips need to remain stable. The feet should remain together as if they've been glued. If you feel one foot moving slightly forward or back during the twist, then you are not stabilizing the hips and pelvis. You need to squeeze everything tighter from the waist down. Drive your sit bones (the two bones under your buttocks) down into the floor and don't let them budge.

- This is another exercise that is great for cleansing the lungs and increasing their capacity. Use the inhalation to fully expand the chest and fill up the lungs. Use the exhalation and twist to push every last drop of air out of the body. Don't forget to keep your mouth shut and breathe only through your nose.

Mother's Little Helper: It's tempting to breeze through this little twist and overlook its enormous benefits when done properly. As you're twisting while lifting your spine (that means no slouching), you can actually whittle away your waist while you relieve pain in your lower back. The twist brings circulation into the hips as well as the mid and lower back area. What people don't realize is that twisting may also aid in digestion as well as possibly energize and massage several organs, including the liver, spleen, and pancreas.[22] According to acupuncturist Ann Cecil-Sterman, "Maintaining pregnancy took a toll on your kidney, spleen and stomach meridians and it is essential that the flow of energy be returned across this region for proper energetic functioning of the body."[23]

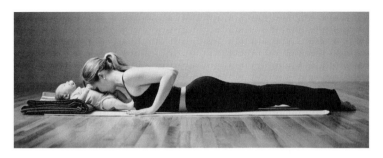

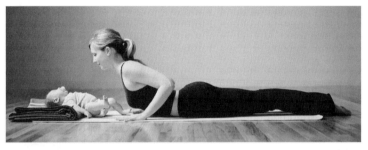

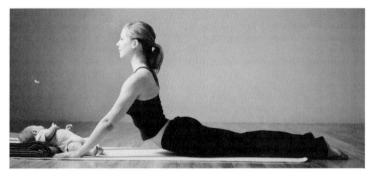

Mom's Placement: Lie flat on your stomach with your chin resting on the floor. Your arms are bent so that your hands are in line with your chest. Press your hands against the floor and pull your elbows in toward your body.

Baby's Placement: Place your baby on your folded blanket (he may be more comfortable propped up on two blankets at an incline). You can choose either to place him on his back looking up at you or on his tummy facing you.

Now What?

1. Spread your fingers out and press your palms deep into the floor.

2. Slide your shoulder blades down toward your tailbone and pull your triceps and elbows tightly into your body. You should already feel your shoulders drawing away from your ears and your collarbone widening across the front of your chest.

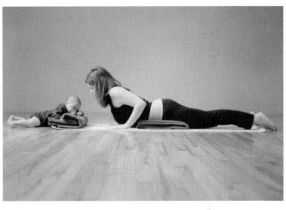

Some women feel uncomfortable lying on their stomachs during their recovery from a C-section, whereas others find this position relaxing. If you are not comfortable, skip this exercise. If you are, place your second folded blanket under your pelvis and lower abdomen to provide gentle padding to your hip bones and the area around your incision. Allow yourself to rise only halfway up; come up just enough to let your chest and shoulders open while keeping the bottom of your rib cage on the mat. Do not arch your lower back.

C - S E C T I O N   T I P

3. Now get your full powerhouse fired up by squeezing your inner thighs together as well as your buttocks, your pelvic floor, and your abdominal wall.

This exercise offers a perfect opportunity to give your baby some active tummy time, something pediatricians strongly recommend. Deliberately placing your baby on his belly can promote a whole cascade of development. Development progresses from the head down. On his stomach, your baby will be more eager to lift his head, which will help him establish head control. Tummy time also encourages your baby to push up on his arms in order to look around and see the world. This builds strength in the arms, back, and neck and increases the muscle tone on the front surface of your baby's body, preparing him to roll over from the stomach to the back, and later to sit, crawl, and begin to walk. Unfortunately, not all babies are enamored of tummy time; in fact, your baby may downright hate it. Try to sneak it in wherever you can, if only for a few moments.

PeeWee Perspective

4. As you inhale, begin to rise up (like a cobra). Start by lifting your head and then expand your chest by pulling your shoulders down away from your ears. Keep pressing your hands into the floor as you continue to lift the front of your torso off the mat.

5. As you exhale, begin to lower back down to the floor. Keep pulling your elbows into your body and drawing your shoulder blades down, like a bird folding its wings.

6. Repeat three to five times.

How Do You Know If You're Doing It Correctly?

- It is important not to crank your neck back or allow your head to fall backward. This is a very common mistake. Keeping your neck long and your chin and gaze level with the horizon will help you avoid strain. Let your head float lightly on top of your cervical spine like a marionette held up by a string.

- How high you should lift up is a personal call; it should be a height that feels challenging but does not compromise your form. If you feel any pain or pinching in your low back, you have gone too high and need to readjust to a height that is appropriate to your comfort level.

- Use your hands to intentionally push the floor away from you rather than letting the weight of your body sit heavily on your hands. Puff up your chest like a pigeon or a seated cat. Try to broaden your shoulders and pull them down and away from your ears.

Mother's Little Helper: How's your posture? Many people believe that just sticking your boobs out and arching your back qualifies as sexy, good posture. What it really does is disengage your stomach and leave you with back pain. One of the true secrets to good posture is strength between your shoulder blades and flexibility across your chest muscles. The cobra is a perfect way to correct slouchy posture and rounded shoulders (kyphosis). It also helps tone the muscles in the back of the upper arms (triceps)—the ones that keep waving even after you've stopped!

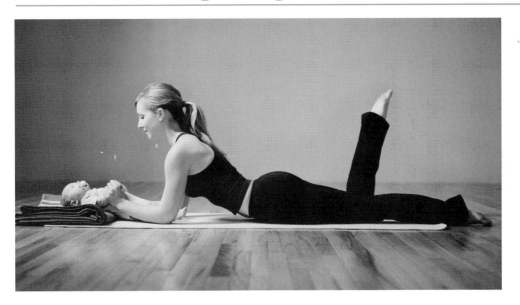

Mom's Placement: Lie on your tummy, propped up on your forearms, facing your little one.

Baby's Placement: Lay your baby on a folded blanket so that she is propped up at a slight incline on her tummy. Her face should be able to peer right into yours.

Now What?

1. Align your shoulders directly above your elbows. Form a light fist with your hands. Gently press your fists and forearms against the floor.
2. Pull your shoulder blades down to expand and lift your chest.
3. Pull your navel up into your spine so that your tummy does not touch the floor. Make sure to curl your tailbone down so that there's no arch in your lower back.
4. Squeeze your butt and squeeze your legs together.
5. Kick your right foot in twice quickly, trying to tap your butt. Then switch and do the same with your left leg.

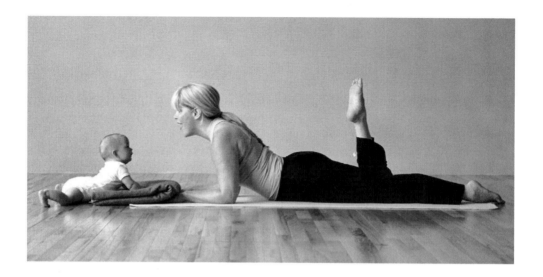

How Do You Know If You're Doing It Correctly?

- Your stomach should not touch the floor and your back should not be arched.
- Push your forearms down, as if you're trying to push the floor down away from you.

Mother's Little Helper: Remember the old saying "If you want to lose five pounds in five seconds, stand up straight and suck in your guts"? Not only does a saggy tummy look sloppy, but it can actually perpetuate pain in your lower back. By holding your stomach off the floor, you begin to lengthen out the extreme arch in your sacrum and protect it from further decompression, pinching, and fusion.

Again we raise the topic of tummy time—not because we're obsessed but because we think it's that important for your younger baby. Tummy time doesn't just give your baby a developmental nudge. It also can help soothe your baby if he has gas or colic. According to prominent New York City acupuncturist Ann Cecil-Sterman, daily tummy time "massages the intestines and keeps the digestive tract in motion."[24]

PeeWee Perspective

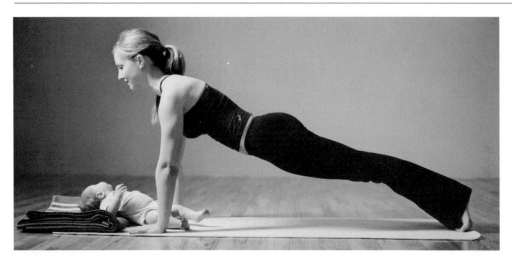

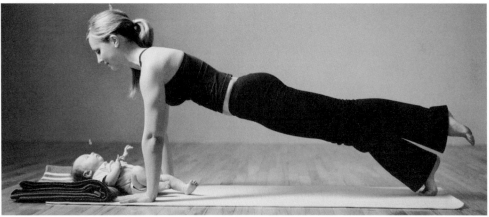

Mom's Placement: Lift your body off the floor with your hands and feet so that you are in a classic push-up or "plank" position. Your hands should line up directly under your shoulders (remember, no wider than your frame), and your back should stay long and straight, with the tailbone gently pulling down to avoid arching in the lower back. Stand on the balls of your feet with your knees straight. Keep your feet slightly separated, no more than the width of your hip bones.

Baby's Placement: Place your folded blanket just ahead of where your hands will be pressing the floor. Rest your baby on his back with his legs between your hands. His head should be at least a few inches past your hands so that he can comfortably look up at you. As another option, you can also put your baby on his tummy, far enough away from your body so that he can look up at you.

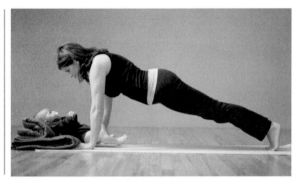

You may do this without the movement in the legs as long as you don't have any discomfort. Just come up into the plank position and hold for five slow breaths. Rest and repeat a few more times. Over time, try to build on the number of breaths you can take while holding this position.

Now What?

1. Inhale as you lift your right leg a few inches straight up off the mat. Then place it back down.
2. Exhale as you do the same with the left leg.
3. Hold your body very still while your legs are moving.
4. Do five to ten sets.

With your baby right below you watching your lips move, you have a nice opportunity to engage in a face-to-face conversation together. By conversing, we're not suggesting you debate the state of child care in this country or some other hot topic; we mean simply using language, nonsensical sounds, and facial expressions, especially your eyes and mouth, to communicate with your baby. Try to take turns, pausing for your baby to respond to you after you say something. Comment about what you see him doing (e.g., "Are you smiling at me?"). If you find yourself saying the same things over and over again, don't worry about boring your baby; he delights in repetition. Try to speak clearly, enunciating your words. Don't be afraid to use baby talk or parentese; remember that your baby actually senses that this special speech is addressed just to him. In the end, don't forget that the amount of talking that you do with your baby has a huge impact on his language development.

PeeWee Perspective

How Do You Know If You're Doing It Correctly?

- Make sure you assume a strong stance throughout your body. Tighten the muscles of the arms, legs, torso, and buttocks to the bones. Just holding this position with intention should be a real challenge!

- Look slightly forward (at your baby), and keep the line from the top of your head all the way to your heels straight and active. Drive the energy back into the heels by pulling the muscles of the legs into the bones and straightening the knees from the back of the knee joints.

- Your body should be one straight line. Do not let your bottom stick up in the air or droop down toward the mat.

- To avoid feeling overwhelmed and heavy in this position, pull your body weight up and press down with your hands and feet. Lift out of your arms and wrists; push the floor away from you rather than expecting it to magically hold you up.

- It is imperative that your powerhouse stay fully engaged to protect your lower back. Don't overdo it. If you feel as if you can't hold it, stop and rest in Child's Pose (see p. 152), and then try again.

Mother's Little Helper: This is a great example of a "weight-bearing" exercise. Who cares? Every woman should, especially postpartum women over thirty. Bone density can decrease for up to six months in lactating mothers.[25]

The good news is that you don't have to grunt through a workout with dumbbells to qualify for resistance training. Weight-bearing exercise includes anything that requires your muscles and bones (muscular-skeletal system) to support the weight of your body against gravity. As you walk around carrying your baby, pushing his stroller, and swinging him around for fun, you are lowering your chances for osteoporosis, arthritis, and fractures resulting from weak spine, hips, and arms.

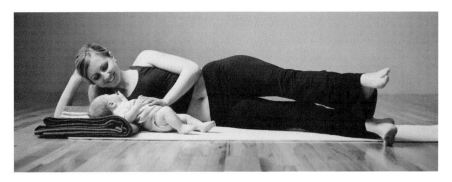

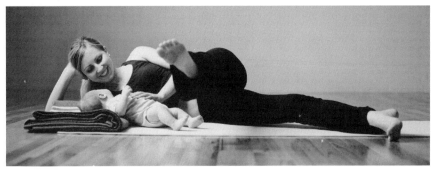

Mom's Placement: Lie down on your right side with your legs extended at about a forty-five-degree angle slightly forward of your hips. To check your position, make sure that you line your trunk up with the back edge of your mat and reach your feet to the forward corner of the mat. Bend your right elbow and prop your head on your hand.

If this bothers your neck, extend your arm fully on the mat and lay your head down on your arm as a pillow.

Baby's Placement: Lay your baby down on his back on a folded blanket in front of your chest area.

Now What?

1. Place your left hand lightly on your baby's tummy or on the floor beside him. Pull your left elbow into your body for stability, and draw your shoulder blades together and down behind your back.
2. Pull your navel to your spine and tighten up the powerhouse.

3. Lift your right leg up to a height that is level with your hip width. To determine this distance, take your hand and find the bone on the front side of your right hip. Don't overestimate this distance and lift your leg too high; your hips are not as wide as you might imagine! While you're lifting your leg, turn your top leg out from the hip joint down to your foot.

Lay your head on your shoulder instead of propping it up with your hand. You can do the leg swing going forward gently, but do not kick your leg back.

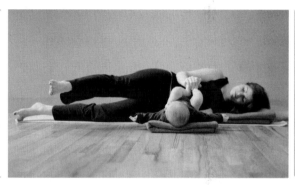

C-SECTION TIP

4. As you exhale, swing your leg forward for two counts. The first count is a strong kick forward in front of you. The second count continues from where the last kick ended with a pulse further forward. Think, "Forward, further forward, and then back." Make sure you don't kick the baby!

5. As you inhale, swing your leg back behind you for one count. Don't extend too far, though, or you'll compromise your form. The hips

Mother's Little Helper: Over the past twenty-five years or so, women's disgust about their thighs has become a national epidemic. Although we feel confident that this exercise can help you strengthen and tone your thigh muscles, we are less hopeful that you are suddenly going to fall in love with your thighs no matter how they turn out. Unfortunately, whenever we harbor insecurity about our own deeper sense of self, we are likely to take this out on our bodies, especially in the form of loathing particular body parts. Joan Jacobs Brumberg, author of *The Body Project,* put it another way: "When an American woman dislikes her thighs, she is unlikely to like herself." "Thunder thighs," she declared, is "shorthand for female anxiety."[26]

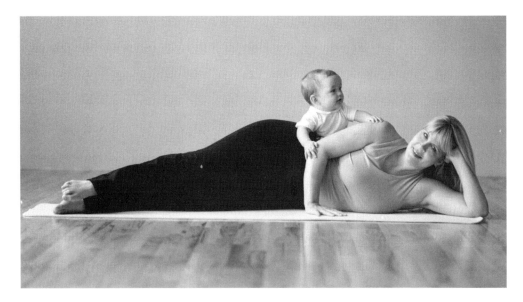

should remain stacked on top of each other and do not roll forward or backward. Use your powerhouse to keep your torso stabilized. Your shoulders and chest should also remain totally still.

6. Repeat up to ten times.

How Do You Know If You're Doing It Correctly?

• Though the side kicks entail moving your leg, what they are actually challenging is the powerhouse. The trick is to keep the rest of your

Using her mom as a jungle gym, Charly is showing off her newly developed motor skills. As babies gain increased mastery over their body movements, they are ever more eager to exercise these new abilities and find new and improved ways to explore their environment. After six months of age, with the acquisition of increased control over his trunk, arms, and legs, your baby can begin to sit up, crawl, and eventually stand. These motor developments give him a whole new perspective on the world and grant him expanding opportunities for autonomy. For example, once your baby can sit up (usually by about eight or nine months), he can turn his head around and look in whatever direction he chooses. No longer is he limited to the view presented from whatever position his mother has opted to put him in.[27]

PeeWee Perspective

body totally still as your leg swings. If you have trouble keeping still, kick your leg with a little less force and range. Control your movements by concentrating on the form.

- Move your legs slowly and gracefully. You're not trying to knock over a cow!

- Keep your leg and ankle long and straight. Try not to grip your front thigh muscle (quadriceps) or lock your knee joint. Don't flex or point your foot; keep it long and loose as if you're moving underwater.

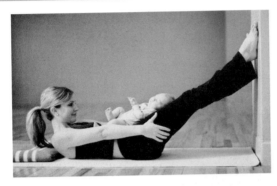
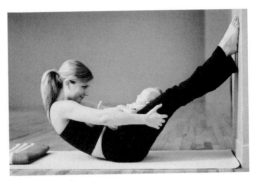
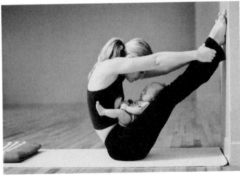

Mom's Placement: Place the front edge of your mat against a wall. Lie on your back with your feet resting against the wall at a forty-five-degree angle. Rest your head on your folded blanket.

Baby's Placement: Sit your baby against your pelvis with his back and head leaning against your thighs.

Now What?

1. Hold your hands around the outer edges of your thighs. Try to keep your shoulders away from your ears and your elbows wide.
2. As you inhale, slowly lift your head forward off the blanket and curl your chin toward your chest.
3. As you exhale, start to roll up, peeling the spine off the mat as you use your hands to gently climb up your legs. Try to go all the way up until your hands reach your ankles.
4. Inhale once you get there, and give your baby a big sloppy kiss!

5. Exhale as you slowly climb your hands down your legs and roll your spine back down to the mat one vertebra at a time.

6. Repeat five to ten times.

C - S E C T I O N   T I P

Instead of putting your legs on the wall, bend your knees and press your toes against the wall. Start by sitting up instead of flat on your back. Hold your hands behind your knees and start to slowly roll down by pulling your navel to your spine and curling your tailbone under. Hollow out the front of your body as you release one vertebra at a time. Let your hands gently slide

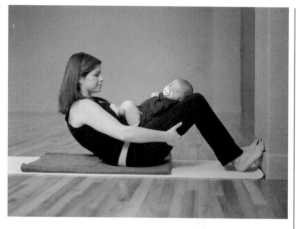

down to help control your roll-down. Once you get about halfway down the spine, work your way back up in the same manner. Work this way until you can go all the way down and up without leaning to either side or jerking to pull yourself up.

How Do You Know If You're Doing It Correctly?

- Make sure your legs are at the right angle for you to roll up. If you're really struggling, you may need to lower your legs a couple of inches so that the angle is less sharp. Pull your navel to your spine to activate your C curve, and reach the crown of your head toward the wall as you

Part of the fun with your baby is teasing him. As you attempt to animate and excite your baby, you naturally tend to inject drama and suspense into the play. While interacting with your baby, think about how often you might make a look of exaggerated, mock surprise on your face, as if something extraordinary just happened. This can really get his juices going. Just remember that babies prefer just enough stimulation to keep them interested; although too little can be boring, too much can disorganize and overwhelm them.

PeeWee Perspective

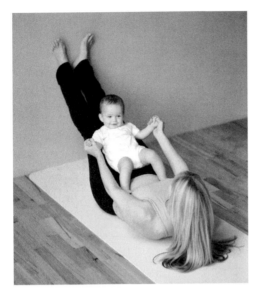 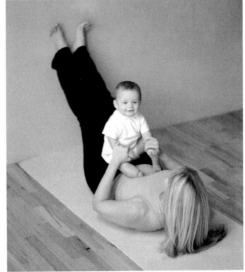

roll up. Be sure you don't lean to either side or use jerky movements.
Use slow, steady control and keep your movements smooth.

- Be patient! This really is as hard as it seems. Rumor has it that Joe Pilates named this exercise The Teaser because the people he assigned
  it to would struggle and laugh, saying, "You've got to be kidding me!"

Mother's Little Helper: Since we're coming to the wall for this exercise, we want to remind you of its utility in case you have to stop working out to feed your baby. If you do
need to take a break, this is no excuse to slump over and hunch your shoulders while feed-
ing your baby. You'll ruin all that good posture you were just working on. Why not keep
the integrity of your Pilates alignment by taking your two folded blankets to the wall and
sitting on them in a cross-legged position and letting the wall support your lower back?

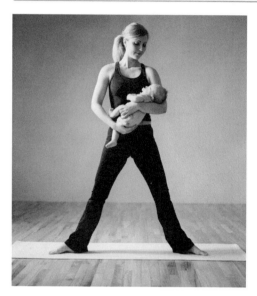 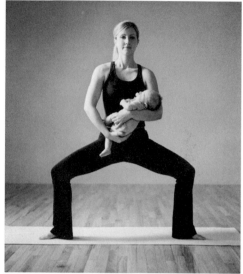

Mom's Placement: Stand on your mat with your feet at least as wide apart as your shoulders. Make sure your legs and feet are turned out from the hips. If you've ever taken ballet, you'll know this as second position.

Baby's Placement: This depends upon your baby's age. Hold a younger baby chest to chest against you or cradled in your arms, providing head and neck support. Let an older baby face outward, and cradle him under his bottom with one arm, bringing your other arm in front of his abdomen.

Now What?

1. Stand with your legs straight and your navel pulled in tight toward your spine.
2. As you exhale, slowly bend your knees out to the side. Bend as low as you can comfortably go, making sure that your knees don't go beyond the line of your ankle.
3. As you inhale, slowly straighten your legs up to start again.
4. Repeat up to ten times.

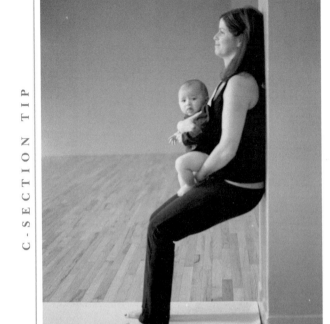

Stand with your back against a wall. Take your feet a few inches away from the wall while your back is supported flat against it. Your feet will remain parallel, with your knees held tightly together. Now slowly bend your knees and slide your back down the wall until you have a ninety-degree angle from your hips to your feet. You should feel as if you are sitting on an invisible chair. Hold this position for about five breaths while you continue pressing your entire spine into the wall. Repeat three times, and try to hold this position for increasing lengths of time, working up to ten breaths.

How Do You Know If You're Doing It Correctly?

- Squeeze your tush and your inner thighs tightly, especially on the way up! Pinch your butt cheeks together as you straighten your legs.

Not all intimate contact with your baby has to be face-to-face. Although babies certainly benefit from direct reciprocal interactions, they also can enjoy being held or cuddled as their caretakers go about their business. T. Berry Brazelton reports that in many different cultures, such as Korea and Japan, young babies are carried around all day by their mothers as they attend to their household duties. In the highlands of Mexico, Brazelton discovered that "mothers rarely, if ever interact with a baby face to face. But they carry the baby in a serape all day long. They breast-feed the baby up to 70–90 times a day. That's being there for the baby!"[28] Enjoy this exercise knowing that your baby is hanging around with you.

PeeWee Perspective

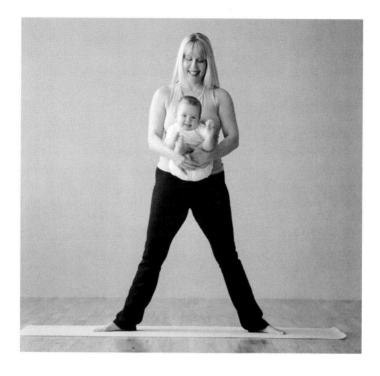

- Imagine that you have a steel rod going down your spine from the top of your head down to your coccyx, or tailbone. Don't arch your lower back or stick your tailbone out. Draw your tailbone slightly under to keep a long line through your spine.

Mother's Little Helper: Notice how Sydney, on page 143, is holding little Evan in her left arm. Though she had no idea she was doing this, her own inclination to favor her left side actually encouraged her son to look up at her face. Infants instinctually prefer to turn their heads to the right, and mothers from many cultures instinctively tend to hold their babies on their left side, creating a perfect harmony.[29] This is just one of the many ways in which a mother's attuned responses to her baby are often second nature. Researchers have called this tendency "intuitive parenting."[30] Another common example of intuitive parenting is the natural tendency to speak in "baby talk" or "parentese." This high-pitched, exaggerated, singsong speech, it turns out, is exactly what appeals most to babies and encourages their own speech development. Isn't it a relief to know that your own intuition can be so on target!

chapter 9

Aches, Pains, and Other Mommy Woes
Remedies Beyond PeeWee Pilates

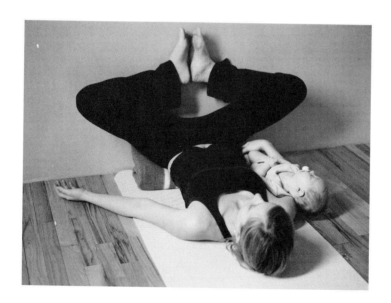

To recover from the strains of pregnancy, childbirth, and early parenting, you need all the help you can get. In this section, we have included some additional movements and postures that target specific postpartum maladies. These movements combine Pilates with restorative yoga.

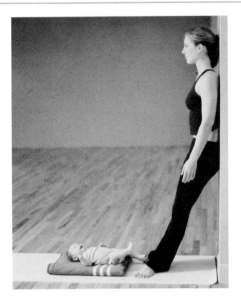 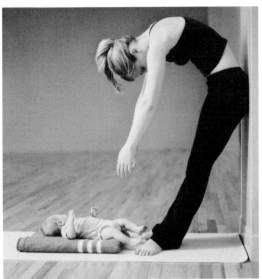

What Is It? This is a classic Pilates exercise done at the wall. Traditionally it is done at the end of the workout to realign the spine so that you walk out of your Pilates session with "perfect" posture.

Who Needs It? Everyone, especially if you have tension in your neck, shoulders, and upper back. This exercise is helpful in teaching you how to isolate each vertebra when rolling up and down the spine.

Mom's Placement: Stand at the wall with your feet in Pilates stance. Place your entire spine (top of the head to the tailbone) against the wall. Be sure that there is no air space between your back and the wall. In order to prevent this, you must engage the powerhouse by squeezing the inner thighs and pelvic floor (how about another Kegel!), pulling the navel to the spine and drawing the rib cage deep into the body. Make sure that your feet are at least ten to twelve inches away from the wall; this way, you can lean against it without falling forward on the roll down.

Baby's Placement: Take your folded blanket and place it in front of your feet. Lay your baby on her back looking up at you.

Now What?

1. Find your position at the wall and let your arms hang heavy from your shoulders.

2. You will roll your spine off the wall one vertebra at a time. Start by dropping your chin down onto your chest, and let the weight of your head pull you down slowly. Be sure you articulate each vertebra without skipping any. Keep your powerhouse engaged, but continue to let your arms hang heavy and your shoulders drop forward like a rag doll.

3. When you reach your sacrum (lower back), stop the roll-down and keep pulling the powerhouse into a C curve.

4. Let your arms become dead weights as your upper body continues to hang heavy.

5. Keeping your arms totally unengaged, let the dead weight hanging from your arms begin to draw floppy, sloppy circles naturally. Don't force them. Feel the weight of your upper back and shoulders fall open across the width of your back. Let the weight of your head release your neck. Imagine that your arms are separated from your shoulder joints. Your arms and upper back should feel loose and droopy.

6. Reverse the circles.

7. Tuck your tailbone under and begin to roll back up the wall. Place one vertebra on the wall at a time. Try to make an imprint of your spine on the wall by pulling the front of your body into the back.

Your baby may be captivated by the movement in your arms. They'll be circling right over her face like a human mobile.

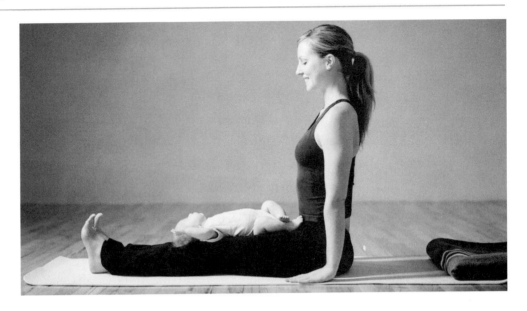

What Is It? This is a standard posture in yoga (dandasana) that is excellent for activating the muscles of the pelvic floor and finding the powerhouse. It is also recommended for poor posture and low back pain.

You may do this on your mat, or you can sit against a wall for extra support.

Who Needs It? We think this is a great posture for everyone, especially for those mothers with low back pain and rounded shoulders. It also helps build strength in that traumatized pelvic floor.

Mom's Placement: Sit up straight with your legs extended in front of you. Take your folded blanket and put it under your sit bones if you find it difficult to sit up with a straight spine or if your lower back feels tender. The blanket will prop you up so that your hips are slightly higher than your knees.

Baby's Placement: Lay your baby on your thighs facing you. If your baby is a little older, you can lay him horizontally across your thighs on his tummy.

Now What?

1. Place your hands on the floor right beside your hips. Press your palms down strongly into the mat, and lift your fingertips off the mat. (You may bend your elbows slightly in toward your waist if you like.) Notice how your shoulder blades activate and pull down while your chest puffs up and your muscles open and expand across your clavicle.

2. Lengthen the back of your neck by reaching your chin down to touch your chest. Keeping your upper body activated in this way, now focus on your lower body.

3. With your legs parallel, flex your feet powerfully by pulling your toes toward your knees. As you do this, your heels may even raise off the mat. As you work your way up your legs, feel your inner thighs pulling into each other and drawing energy up into your pelvic floor.

4. Squeeze your pelvic floor and buttocks so that you feel yourself sitting on top of the floor instead of sinking down into it.

5. Imagine you're wearing an ultratight pair of jeans and you don't want your belly to pooch out. Pull your navel back into your spine and up under your rib cage. (Not a physical possibility, we know, but it's a good visual.)

6. Deflate your rib cage and hug it back toward your spine. Don't let your ribs poke out.

Now hold this posture with full intensity for five slow breaths through your nose. Try to add an extra breath every time until you work up to ten deep breaths.

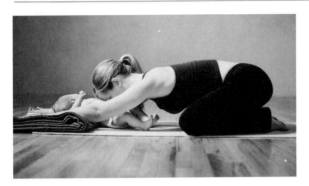 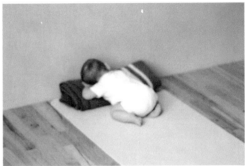

What Is It? This is one of the most common restorative or resting poses in yoga asana. It is often used in yoga classes as a sort of "rest stop" during vigorous practice because it can help regulate the heart rate and blood pressure. It is also considered a very introspective pose since the head and heart are recoiled into themselves rather than opening out into the world. It is a nice position for meditation when you feel you have spread yourself too thin and need to regroup or gather your thoughts.

Who Needs It? We'll go out on a limb again here and say, "Everyone"—but specifically people with low back pain, sciatica, tension in the neck, high blood pressure, and stress.

Mom's Placement: With the tops of your feet on the floor, sit back on your heels, with your knees open as wide as your hips. (Your feet should touch each other.) Stretch your arms forward on the mat, pressing your stomach into your thighs and releasing your head down between your arms. Your forehead should be resting against the mat.

Baby's Placement: Place your baby on her blanket flat on her back. The blanket should be right in front of you, within your reach.

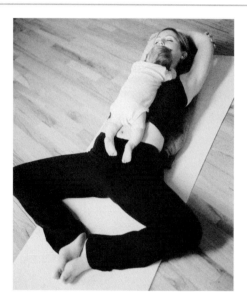

What Is It? This is another restorative posture from yoga. With your chest open, this position suggests an opening of your heart chakra and is considered more rejuvenating than the more introverted and self-reflective Child's Pose.

Who Needs It? We hate to sound repetitious but—everyone. It is especially good for those suffering from depression and low energy. It is also recommended for posture issues, shoulder pain, neck pain, and back pain and for women who are breast-feeding.

Mom's Placement: Stack both of your blankets folded into quarters on top of each other on your mat. Roll them into one long Tootsie Roll shape to create a bolster. Sit in front of the narrow end of the Tootsie Roll. Your sacrum should be touching the tip of the roll. Now lay your spine right on top of the length of the roll. Let the roll encourage your chest to open.

Make the shape of a diamond with your legs. Bend your knees and let them fall open to the side while you gently press the soles of your feet together. You may hold your baby (with one arm) facing you on your chest or cradle him in one arm beside you. Do whatever works for you here. If your baby does not need the support, let your arms stretch back over your head and lightly pull your elbows with your opposite hands (a lovely extra stretch for the chest and shoulders). Close your eyes and relax. In our experience, this posture is very comforting and reassuring to most babies and may lure yours into sleep.

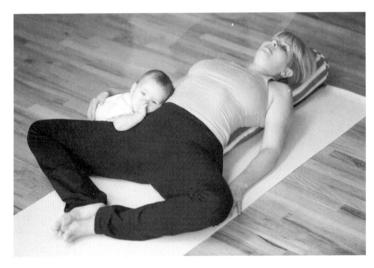

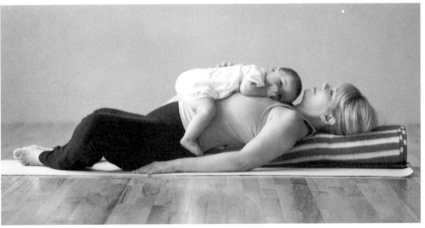

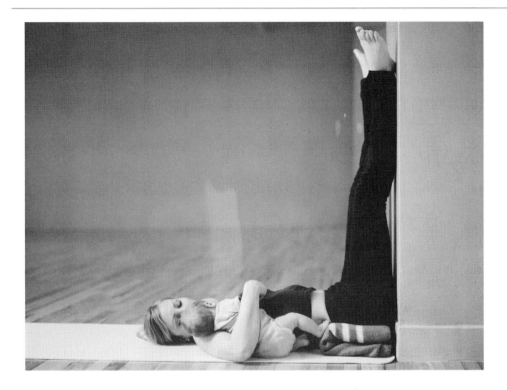

What Is It? The Wall Tower is a gentle, restorative variation on the Tower, a classic Pilates exercise performed on the Cadillac. (The Cadillac is a type of Pilates equipment.) This posture releases the lower back and hamstrings and increases circulation in the legs and feet.

Who Needs It? This is especially good for relieving pain or stiffness in the lower back. It is also good for those with tight hamstrings, swollen ankles and feet, and high blood pressure.

Mom's Placement: Take your two folded blankets and stack them on top of each other against a wall. Lie down with your butt on top of the blankets and your legs resting up against the wall a few inches apart. Try to press your sit bones deep into the wall and relax your hip flexors.

Baby's Placement: You can hold your baby in any way you choose here. It is nice to cradle her in one of your arms resting on the floor or let her lie on your chest. Many babies remain quite content with you here.

Now close your eyes and try to relax deeper into the position for five or ten minutes (baby permitting).

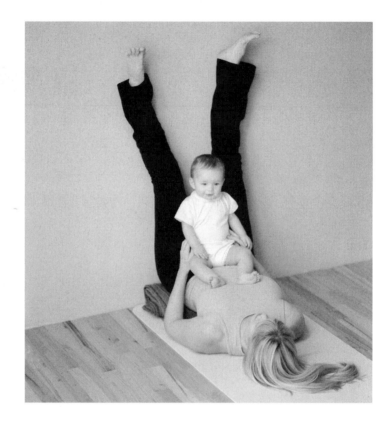

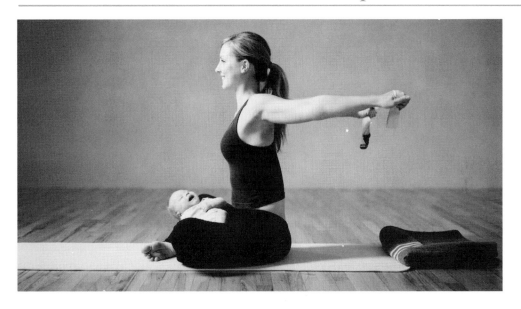

What Is It? This is a simple stretch to open and release the shoulders and chest. Grab a yoga strap or Thera-Band. (If you don't have either, you can use a medium-sized towel or even an old pair of pantyhose!)

Who Needs It? This is a great relief when you have tension in your upper back, chest, or shoulders. Also it can do wonders for slouchy posture. We recommend it especially for women who are breast-feeding, stressed, or dealing with postpartum depression.

Mom's Placement: You can do this seated in a cross-legged position or standing.

Baby's Placement: Place your baby near you in a comfortable position on the blanket.

Now What?

1. Hold your yoga strap with your hands in a wide position and your arms stretched out in front of you.

2. Slowly reach your arms up over your head and take them as far as you can behind you. Do not let your elbows bend or your shoulders lift. Pull your shoulder blades down so that your arms can rotate in your shoulder joints.

3. Take your arms back up and over to the front.

4. Repeat up to ten times.

As your shoulders start to loosen up, try to bring your hands a little bit closer together on the strap. Notice how much more stretch you get as the space between the hands narrows. Just be sure you don't overdo it. If you move your hands too close together, your shoulders will lift and your elbows will bend.

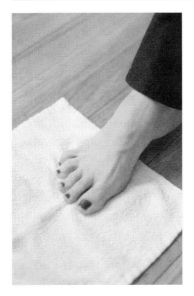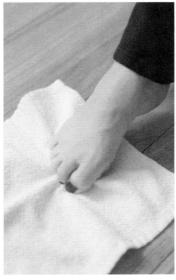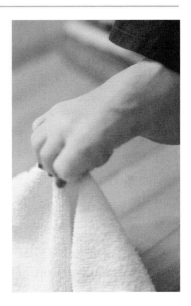

What Is It? This is a simple exercise to strengthen, stretch, and improve circulation in the feet and toes.

Who Needs It? If you are having any discomfort or weakness in your feet, this is a great help. It's also good for fallen arches, swelling in the feet and ankles, and problems with balance.

Mom's Placement: You can choose to either sit in a chair or stand. (Keep in mind that standing requires more balance.) Spread your towel out on the floor in front of one foot.

Baby's Placement: Place him on his blanket near you. Just be sure he's not too close to you if you're standing, so that you don't accidentally step on him if you lose your balance!

Now What?

1. Place your foot flat on the towel.
2. Start by flexing your foot and lifting all of your toes off the floor. Leave the ball of your foot down on the towel.
3. Keeping your toes up, separate and spread them out like a fan.

4. Now think of your toes as your fingers. Place them down on the towel one at a time starting with the pinky toe. Articulate each toe and notice if any of them don't want to go down alone.
5. Once all toes are down, grip the towel with your toes.
6. Pull the towel back toward you by curling your toes back and under.
7. Repeat three times. Keep pulling the towel farther back to you.
8. After the third pull, hold the towel in your toe grip and try to lift it off the floor without dropping it.
9. Repeat five times with each foot.

We believe that strong, flexible feet just might be the key to happiness. Don't neglect or underestimate them. After all, they are the platform that you stand on, and they carry you wherever you walk, run, or dance in life. If your feet have a problem, it is almost sure to create more problems somewhere else in your body.

Acknowledgments

We would first like to thank our agent, Debra Goldstein, who, as a hot new mama herself, immediately embraced our idea, kept our feet on the ground, and led us to a home at Da Capo Press. We would also like to thank Nicole Austin and everyone else at The Creative Culture who helped us so kindly along the way.

We couldn't have asked for a more supportive, accessible editor than Marnie Cochran (despite her unfortunate affinity for the Red Sox). Thanks for remaining calm and nurturing us through our infantile moments of panic, hysteria, and adult-onset colic.

Thank you, too, to Erin Sprague, our project editor, for your careful review.

We lucked out with Jonathan Pozniak (JPoz) as our patient, hard-working, saintly photographer. You've been a Godsend and a true talent. Thank you for bringing this book to life!

An especially huge thanks goes to our beautiful model moms and their adorable babies: Kasey and Charly Gittleman, Sydney and Evan Holly, and Cathy and Kyle Malin. You were all such a privilege and pleasure to work with, as well as an inspiration to us.

We are enormously grateful for the wisdom, insight, and generous time offered by our two consulting physicians, Dr. Shereen Russell and Dr. Natalie Geary. We would also like to thank Dr. Amy Lewis and Ann Cecil-Sturman for their helpful input.

An additional thanks goes out to Alexis Stewart, who so generously allowed us to photograph in her stunning, tranquil studio. Many thanks as well to Be Yoga/YogaWorks Westside for granting us access to their studio space.

Holly:

First I want to thank my incredible family for their constant love, support, and humor.

I am forever in awe of my teachers: Romana Kryzanowska and Bob Liekens. Thank you for your mastery, integrity, and spirit. You've kept me on my toes and your voices have never left my head.

I am immensely grateful to the creators of Baby Om, Sarah Perron and Laura Staton. Your training taught me more than I could have imagined. Namaste to both of you!

To Ron Teitlebaum, thank you for giving me a new start.

Thank you Alexis Stewart for the freedom you gave me to develop this idea.

To Bob Murphy, thank you for allowing me to continue my work and helping it grow.

I have been blessed with the most awesome clients in New York City. I appreciate your patience and support during this process. I love you all like kittens and you look fabulous!

To my friends who keep me in line and laughing: Kim Crutcher, Adam McLaughlin, Donna Jane Gentile, Carrie Lenehan, Jerre Dye, Monique Harrington, Paddy Mullen, Carmen Kelsey, Craig and Chris Benelli, Andrew Hall, and Ron Haney.

Love to my sweet potato, Niall Slevin. I look forward to our own tater tot someday.

Thank you Zoe and Jonas for letting me take your mother hostage. I owe you big time.

And finally, to my supermodel coauthor Stacy. Thank you would never be enough to express my gratitude for all of the fantastic work you've done. I appreciate the sacrifices you made taking this on, and I'm happy to call you my business partner as well as my dear friend.

Stacy:

When I started Pilates a number of years ago to get rid of my terrible slouch, I never anticipated that it would lead to anything beyond a slightly straighter spine. Now, after years of working with Holly, I am thankful not only for my own improved posture, but also for the opportunity to work together to create PeeWee Pilates and launch this book. Holly, thank you so much for trusting me, forcing me to write, entertaining me with your offbeat humor, offering up your friendship, and overall kicking my butt!

Zoe and Jonas, you two were my favorite teachers about infant development. Zoe, I want to thank you for reading revisions over and over without ever protesting and for rendering your very excellent suggestions. Jonas, I want to thank you for being so patient with me and for forgoing playtime in the park and chess games so I could work. And Jacky Umali, you deserve a medal for taking care of all of us.

There ain't nothing like great friends. Rebecca Drill, Randi Roth, and Wendy Brandes, thank you so much for taking the time—when you've had so little to spare—to read through the manuscript and offer your feedback with such diplomacy. A huge thanks, too, to Risa Ribakove, Meg Kaplan, and Daniel Weitzman for your nonstop encouragement and caring.

I am also grateful to Doris Silverman, for her insights in development and her persistent reassurances, and to my mentor, Philip Bromberg, who encouraged me to "reach for the moon." And Willa Cobert, how lucky I am that you're always in my court.

Cathy Malin, I adore you and am so glad that you chose to have Kyle when you did. Kyle, I can't wait until you're old enough to check yourself out and chuckle. To Hope and Herb Malin and to Robin and Jason Rubinstein. What would I do without you?

And a big love to Steven Katz, my Fairfield boy, and to the new PeeWees in my life, Max, Zoe, and Haley.

Notes

Introduction

1. Thomas F. Cash, "A Negative Body Image," in Thomas F. Cash and Thomas Pruzinsky (Eds.), *Body Image: A Handbook of Theory, Research, and Clinical Practice*, Guilford Press, 2002, pp. 269–276.

2. L. Smolak, *Next Door Neighbors Puppet Guide Book*, National Eating Disorders Association, 1996.

3. See, for example, Daniel Stern, *The Interpersonal World of the Infant*, Basic Books, 1985; Stanley Greenspan with Nancy Breslau Lewis, *Building Healthy Minds*, Da Capo Press, 1999; and Daniel J. Siegel, *The Developing Mind: How Relationship and the Brain Interact to Shape Who We Are*, Guilford Press, 1999.

Chapter 1: Potbell and All

1. Sandy Jones and Marcie Jones, *Great Expectations: Your All-in-One Resource for Pregnancy and Childbirth*, Barnes & Noble, 2004, p. 284.

2. Dawnine Enette Larson-Meyer, "Effect of Postpartum Exercise on Mothers and Their Offspring: A Review of the Literature," *Obesity Research*, Vol. 10, pp. 841–853, 2002.

3. Mary L. O'Toole, Marjorie A. Sawicki, and Raul Artal, "Structured Diet and Physical Activity Prevent Postpartum Weight Retention," *Journal of Women's Health*, Vol. 12, No. 10, pp. 991–998, 2003.

4. Michael G. Perri, A. Martin, A. Daniel, Elizabeth A. Leermakers, Samuel F. Sears, et al., "Effects of Group- Versus Home-Based Exercise in the Treatment of Obesity," *Journal of Consulting and Clinical Psychology*, Vol. 65, No. 2, pp. 278–285, 1997.

5. Erika Ringdahl, "Promoting Postpartum Exercise," *Physician and Sports Medicine*, Vol. 30, No. 2, pp. 31–36, 2002.

6. Laura Staton and Sarah Perron, *Baby Om*, Henry Holt, 2002, p. 232.

7. I. Nygaard, J. O. DeLancey, L. Arnsdorf, and E. Murphy, "Exercise and Incontinence," *Obstetrics and Gynecology,* Vol. 75, pp. 848–885, 1990.

8. Theresa Francis-Cheung, *Pregnancy Weight Management,* Adams Media, 2000.

9. Ann Douglas, *The Mother of All Baby Books,* Wiley, 2002.

10. Based on a review of a study titled the First National Health and Nutrition Examination Survey (NHANES) in Larson-Meyer, op. cit.

11. Ringdahl, op. cit.

12. O'Toole, Sawicki, and Artal, op. cit.

13. Marvin S. Eiger and Sally Wendkos Olds, *The Complete Book of Breastfeeding,* 3rd ed., Workman Publishing, 1999.

14. Francis-Cheung, op. cit.

15. Larson-Meyer, op. cit.

16. T. J. Quinn and G. B. Carey, "Does Exercise Intensity or Diet Influence Lactic Acid Accumulation in Breast Milk?" *Medicine and Science in Sports and Exercise,* pp. 105–109, 1999.

17. Jones and Jones, op. cit.

18. Based on discussions with Dr. Sherrell Russell.

Chapter 2: If Mama Ain't Happy

1. According to the American College of Obstetricians and Gynecologists, as cited on www.MayoClinic.com, in a summary on postpartum depression sponsored by the Mayo Foundation for Medical Education and Research.

2. See Ruta M. Nonacs, "Ph.D.'s Overview of Postpartum Depression," on eMedicine Health.com, updated August 8, 2004.

3. See the Web site Depression After Delivery, Inc.: www.depressionafterdelivery.com. It is a national nonprofit organization that provides support for women with postpartum disorders (PPD).

4. For example, see M. K. Weinberg, E. Z. Tronick, M. Beeghly, K. L. Olson, H. Kernan, and J. M. Riley, "Subsyndromal Depressive Symptoms and Major Depression in Postpartum Women," *American Journal of Orthopsychiatry,* Vol. 71, No. 1, pp. 87–97, 2001.

5. See, for example, www.depressionafterdelivery.com, op. cit.

6. See, for example, E. Z. Tronick, "Emotions and Emotional Communication in Infants," *American Psychologist,* Vol. 44, pp. 112–119, 1989, and Harriet Field, "Infants of Depressed Mothers," *Infant Behavior and Development,* Vol. 18, pp. 1–13, 1995.

7. K. F. Koltyn and S. S. Schultes, "Psychological Effects of an Aerobic Exercise Session and a Rest Session Following Pregnancy," *Journal of Sports Medicine and Physical Fitness,* Vol. 37, pp. 287–291, 1997.

8. R. Clark, A. Tluczek, and A. Wenzel, "Psychotherapy for Postpartum Depression: A Preliminary Report," *American Journal of Orthopsychiatry,* Vol. 73, No. 4, pp. 441–454, 2003.

9. Christiane Northrup, *Women's Bodies, Women's Wisdom,* Bantam Books, 1998, p. 746.

10. A. B. Ransjo-Arvidson, E. Nissen, and K. Uvnas-Moberg, "Postpartum Maternal Oxytocin Release by Newborns: Effects of Infant Hand Massage and Sucking," *Birth,* pp. 13–19, 2001.

11. Linda F. Palmer, *Baby Matters: What Your Doctor May Not Tell You About Caring for Your Baby,* Baby Reference, 2004.

12. Sarah Blaffer Hrdy, *Mother Nature: A History of Mothers, Infants, and Natural Selection,* Pantheon, 1999, p. 154. Also quoted in Katherine Ellison, *The Mommy Brain: How Motherhood Makes Us Smarter,* Basic Books, 2005, p. 87.

13. In a personal conversation (June 2005), Dr. Amy B. Lewis, a highly regarded dermatologist in New York City, reported that a patented botanical compound called regenetrol complex has been demonstrated in clinical trials to reduce stretch marks. This active agent is available through a prescription cream.

14. S. H. Fischman, E. A. Rankin, K. L. Soeken, and E. R. Lenz, "Changes in Sexual Relationships in Postpartum Couples," *Journal of Obstetrics, Gynecology, and Neonatal Nursing,* Vol. 15, No. 1, pp. 58–63, 1986.

15. Ibid.

16. See Ann Kearney-Cooke, "Familial Influences on Body Image Development," in Thomas F. Cash and Thomas Pruzinsky (Eds.), *Body Image: A Handbook of Theory, Research and Clinical Practice,* Guilford Press, 2002.

17. Leslie J. Heinberg and Angela S. Guarda, "Body Image Issues in Obstetrics and Gynecology," in Thomas F. Cash and Thomas Pruzinsky (Eds.), *Body Image: A Handbook of Theory, Research and Clinical Practice,* Guilford Press, 2002.

18. Janet Polivy and C. Peter Herman, "If at First You Don't Succeed: False Hopes of Self-Change," *American Psychologist,* Vol. 57, No. 9, pp. 677–689, 2002.

19. D. J. Boardley, R. G. Sargent, A. L. Coker, J. R. Hussey, and P. A. Sharpe, "The Relationship Between Diet, Activity, and Other Factors, and Postpartum Weight Change by Race," *Obstetrics and Gynecology,* Vol. 86, pp. 834–838, 1995.

20. J. Kevin Thompson, Leslie J. Heinberg, Madeline Altabe, and Stacey Tantleff-Dunn, *Exacting Beauty: Theory, Assessment, and Treatment of Body Image Disturbance,* American Psychological Association, 1999.

Chapter 3: Wonderbaby

1. Lise Eliot, *What's Going on in There? How the Brain and Mind Develop in the First Five Years of Life,* Bantam Books, 1999.

2. Ibid.

3. Beverly Stokes, *Amazing Babies: Essential Movement for Your Baby in the First Year,* Move Alive Media, 2002.

4. Phillipe Rochat, *The Infant's World,* Harvard University Press, 2001.

5. Allen N. Schore, *Affect Regulation and the Origin of the Self,* Erlbaum, 1994.

6. Joanna Lipari, "Raising Baby: What You Need to Know," *Psychology Today,* July-August 2000.

7. Eliot, op. cit.

8. Stanley Greenspan with Nancy Breslau Lewis, *Building Healthy Minds,* Da Capo Press, 1999, p. 9.

9. Charles W. Snow and Cindy G. McGah, *Infant Development,* Prentice Hall, 2003.

10. Ibid.

11. See, for example, Beatrice Beebe and Frank M. Lachmann, "Co-Constructing Inner and Relational Processes: Self- and Mutual Regulation in Infant Research and Adult Treatment," *Psychoanalytic Psychology,* Vol. 15, No. 4, pp. 480–516, 1998.

12. See, for example, E. Z. Tronick, "Why Is Connection with Others So Critical? The Formation of Dyadic States of Consciousness: Coherence Governed Selection and the Co-Creation of Meaning Out of Messy Meaning Making," in J. Nadel and D. Muir (Eds.), *Emotional Development,* Oxford University Press, pp. 293–315, 2005; Daniel Stern, *The Interpersonal World of the Infant,* Basic Books, 1985; Joseph Jaffe, Beatrice Beebe, Stanley Feldstein, Cynthia L Crown, and Michael D. Jasnow, *Rhythms of Dialogue in Infancy: Monographs of the Society for Research in Child Development,* Blackwell, 2001; and Daniel J. Siegel, *The Developing Mind,* Guilford Press, 1999.

13. P. Nicely, C. Tamis-LeMonda, and M. Bornstein, "Mothers' Attuned Responses to Infant Affect Expressivity Promote Earlier Achievement of Language Milestones," *Infant Behavior and Development,* Vol. 22, No. 4, pp. 557–568, 1999, and P. Nicely, C. Tamis-LeMonda, and W. Grolnick, "Maternal Responsiveness to Infant Affect: Stability and Prediction," *Infant Behavior and Development,* Vol. 22, No. 1, pp. 103–117, 1999.

14. Esther Thelen, "Motor Development: A New Synthesis," *American Psychologist,* Vol. 50, No. 2, pp. 79–95, 1995.

15. Snow and McGah, op. cit.

16. Eliot, op. cit.

17. Darwin Muir and Alan Slater (Eds.), *Infant Development: The Essential Readings,* Blackwell, 2000, p. 106.

18. Eliot, op. cit.

19. E. Z. Tronick, H. Alz, L. Adamson, S. Wise, and T. B. Brazelton, "The Infant's Response to Entrapment Between Contradictory Messages in Face-to-Face Interaction," *Journal of the American Academy of Child Psychiatry,* Vol. 17, pp. 1–13, 1978.

20. Kathy Hirsh-Pasek and Roberta Michnick Golinkoff with Diane Eyer, *Einstein Never Used Flash Cards: How Our Children REALLY Learn—and Why They Need to Play More and Memorize Less,* Rodale, 2003.

21. See, for example, Marsha Kaitz, Pnina Lapidot, Ruth Bronner, and Arthur I. Eidelman, "Parturient Women Can Recognize Their Infants by Touch," *Developmental Psychology,* Vol. 28, No. 1, pp. 35–39, 1992; K. Grossmann, K. Thane, and K. E. Grossmann, "Maternal Tactual Contact of the Newborn After Various Postpartum Conditions of Mother-Infant Contact," *Developmental Psychology,* Vol. 17, No. 2, pp. 158–169, 1981; and J. Schaller, S. G. Carlsson, and K. Larsson, "Effects of Extended Post-Partum Mother-Child Contact on the Mother's Behavior During Nursing," *Infant Behavior and Development,* Vol. 2, pp. 319–324, 1979.

22. Eliot, op. cit.

23. Ibid., p. 143.

24. Rochat, op. cit.

25. Eliot, op. cit.

26. Hirsh-Pasek and Golinkoff with Eyer, op. cit.

27. Ibid.

28. Eliot, op. cit., p. 367.

29. For example, see C. S. Tamis-LeMonda, M. H. Bornstein, and L. Baumwell, "Maternal Responsiveness and Children's Achievement of Language Milestones," *Child Development,* Vol. 72, No. 3, pp. 748–767, 2001.

30. Muir and Slater, op. cit., p. 242.

31. Hui-Chin Hsu and Alan Fogel, "Social Regulatory Effects of Infant Nondistress Vocalization on Maternal Behavior," *Developmental Psychology,* Vol. 39, No. 6, pp. 976–991, 2003.

32. M. H. Bornstein and C. S. Tamis-LeMonda, "Maternal Responsiveness and Cognitive Development in Children," in M. H. Bornstein (Ed.), *Maternal Responsiveness: Characteristics and Consequences,* New Directions for Child Development No. 43, Jossey-Bass, pp. 49–61, 1989.

33. M. H. Bornstein, C. S. Tamis-LeMonda, S. Tal, P. Ludemann, S. Toda, and C. Rahn, "Maternal Responsiveness to Infants in Three Societies: The United States, France, and Japan," *Child Development,* Vol. 63, pp. 808–821, 1992.

34. Eliot, op. cit.

35. E. Thelen and J. Spencer, "Postural Control During Reaching in Young Infants: A Dynamic Systems Approach," *Neuroscience and Biobehavioral Reviews,* Vol. 22, pp. 507–514, 1998.

36. Eliot, op. cit., p. 289.

37. Snow and McGah, op. cit., p. 109.

38. Rochat, op. cit.

39. C. K. Rovee-Collier, M. W. Sullivan, M. Enright, D. Lucas, and J. W. Fagan, "Reactivation of Infant Memory," *Science,* Vol. 208, pp. 1159–1161, 1980, and C. Rovee-Collier and M. J. Gekoski, "The Economics of Conjugate Reinforcement: A Review of Conjugate

Reinforcement," in H. W. Reese and L. P. Lisitt (Eds.), *Advances in Child Development and Behavior*, Vol. 13, Academic Press, 1979, pp. 195–255.

    40. Thelen, op. cit., p. 91.

Chapter 4: Roll Out Your Mat!

    1. Bess H. Marcus, LeighAnn H. Forsyth, Elaine J. Stone, Patricia M. Dubbert, Thomas L. McKenzie, Andrea L. Dunn, and Steven N. Blair, "Physical Activity Behavior Change: Issues in Adoption and Maintenance," *Health Psychology*, Vol. 19, No. 1S, pp. 32–41, 2000.

Chapter 5: A Crash Course in Pilates

    1. B. K. S. Iyengar, *Light on Yoga*, Schocken Books, 1977, pp. 515–516.

    2. Ibid., p. 43.

Chapter 6: Mommy's Little Powerhouse

    1. Daniel Stern, *Diary of a Baby*, Basic Books, 1998, p. 39.

    2. Susan Ludington-Hoe and Susan K. Golant, *How to Have a Smarter Baby: The Infant Stimulation Program for Enhancing Your Baby's Natural Development*, Bantam Books, 1985.

    3. Ibid.

    4. Laura Staton and Sarah Perron, *Baby Om: Yoga for Mothers and Babies*, Henry Holt, 2002.

    5. Stanley Greenspan with Nancy Breslau Lewis, *Building Healthy Minds*, Da Capo Press, 1999.

    6. Linda Acredolo and Susan Goodwyn, *Baby Minds: Brain-Building Games Your Baby Will Love*, Bantam Books, 2000.

Chapter 8: The PeeWee Pilates Exercises

    1. Christiane Northrup, *Women's Bodies, Women's Wisdom*, Bantam Books, 1998, p. 322.

    2. B. K. S. Iyengar, *Light on Yoga*, Schocken Books, 1977.

    3. Lise Eliot, *What's Going on in There? How the Brain and Mind Develop in the First Five Years of Life*, Bantam Books, 1999, p. 345.

    4. Joseph Jaffe, Beatrice Beebe, Stanley Feldstein, Cynthia L. Crown, and Michael D. Jasnow, *Rhythms of Dialogue in Infancy*, Monographs of the Society for Research in Child Development, Serial No. 265, Vol. 66, No. 2, 2001.

5. Eliot, op. cit.

6. Linda Acredolo and Susan Goodwyn, *Baby Minds: Brain-Building Games Your Baby Will Love*, Bantam Books, 2000, p. 101.

7. Eliot, op. cit.

8. Cheryl J. Hansen, Larry C. Stevens, and Richard J. Coast, "Exercise Duration and Mood State: How Much Is Enough to Feel Better?" *Health Psychology*, Vol. 20, No. 4, pp. 267–275, 2001.

9. A. Meltzoff and M. Moore, "Imitations in Newborns: Exploring the Range of Gestures Imitated and the Underlying Mechanisms," *Developmental Psychology*, Vol. 25, pp. 954–962, 1989.

10. C. Rovee-Collier and H. Hayne, "Memory in Infancy and Early Childhood," in E. Tulving (Ed.*), The Oxford Handbook of Memory*, Oxford University Press, 2002, pp. 267–282.

11. Daphne de Marneffe, *Maternal Desire: On Children, Love and the Inner Life*, Back Bay Books/Little, Brown, 2004, p. 99.

12. Darwin Muir and Alan Slater (Eds.), *Infant Development: The Essential Readings*, Blackwell, 2000.

13. Daniel Stern, *The Motherhood Constellation: A Unified View of Parent-Infant Psychotherapy*, Basic Books, 1995, as reviewed in Douglas Davies, *Child Development*, Guilford Press, 2004, p. 150.

14. Basic Books, 2005.

15. For more detailed information on infant massage, there are several books you might check out. Three that we recommend are Frederick Loboyer, *Loving Hands: The Traditional Art of Baby Massage*, Newmarket Press, 1997; Vimala Schneider McClure, *Infant Massage—Revised Edition: A Handbook for Loving Parents*, Bantam Books, 2000; and Peter Walker, *Baby Massage: A Practical Guide to Massage and Movement for Babies and Infants*, St. Martin's Press, 1996.

16. Uzzi Reiss and Yfat M. Reiss, *How to Make a New Mother Happy*, Chronicle Books, 2004.

17. Phillipe Rochat, *The Infant's World*, Harvard University Press, 2001.

18. Daniel Stern, *Diary of a Baby*, Basic Books, 1990.

19. Stanley Greenspan with Nancy Breslau Lewis, *Building Healthy Minds*, Da Capo Press, 1999, p. 28.

20. Ibid.

21. Daniel N. Stern, "Commentary: Fact-to-Face Play: Its Temporal Structure as Predictor of Socioaffective Development," in *Rhythms of Dialogue in Infancy: Coordinated Timing in Development*, Monographs of the Society for Research in Child Development, Serial No. 265, Vol. 66, No. 2, p. 145, 2001.

22. Iyengar, op. cit.

23. Based on a personal conversation with Holly Jean Cosner.

24. Ibid.

25. Dawnine Enette Larson-Meyer, "Effect of Postpartum Exercise on Mothers and Their Offspring: A Review of the Literature," *Obesity Research*, Vol. 10, pp. 841–853, 2002.

26. Joan Jacobs Brumberg, *The Body Project: An Intimate History of American Girls*, Viking Books, 1997, p. 128.

27. Davies, op. cit.

28. T. Berry Brazelton and Stanley I. Greenspan, *The Irreducible Needs of Children*, Da Capo Press, 2000, pp. 12–13.

29. Doris Silverman, "Attachment Research: An Approach to a Developmental Relational Perspective," in Neil J. Skolnick and Susan C. Warshaw (Eds.), *Relational Perspectives in Psychoanalysis*, the Analytic Press, 1992.

30. H. Papousek and M. Papousek, "Intuitive Parenting: A Dialectic Counterpart to the Infant's Integrative Competence," in Joy Osofsky (Ed.), *Handbook of Infant Development*, 2nd ed., Wiley, 1987, pp. 669–720.

About Our Models

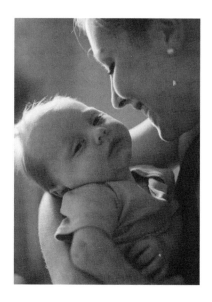

Sydney and Evan

Mom: Sydney, a first-time mom in her early thirties, has worked as a yoga instructor and modern dancer.

Evan: Seven and a half weeks old.

Delivery: Vaginal with no complications.

Started PeeWee Pilates: Six weeks postpartum.

Sydney's impression of PeeWee Pilates: "Even though I did yoga throughout my pregnancy and had a pretty easy delivery, I was frustrated to discover that I couldn't find the strength to do even a single roll-up when I began working with Holly. It looked so simple and yet it's so hard. I completely lost the connection to my midsection. I just couldn't find it. I'm determined now to recover the strength I had before I got pregnant. And I love that I get to hold and cuddle with Evan while I'm exercising. I'm not ready to leave him alone."

Working with Sydney and Evan: Sydney began PeeWee Pilates when Evan was just on the cusp of "waking up to the world."* As a very young infant, he still spent much of his time either asleep or nursing and was not yet actively alert for very long stretches of time. Given his placid state, Sydney was able right away to concentrate on her own form and breathing, while Evan quietly enjoyed nestling into his mama's body. Emphasis was given to ensuring that Evan received adequate neck and back support and was in all ways comfortable and safe. Clearly in the thrall of a love affair with her new son, Sydney seemed to delight in the physical closeness with him throughout the exercises. She couldn't take her eyes off him and kissed him every chance she got. The sessions had a serene, dreamy quality to them and were only interrupted when Evan wanted to nurse.

---

*Phillipe Rochat, *The Infant's World*, Harvard University Press, 2001.

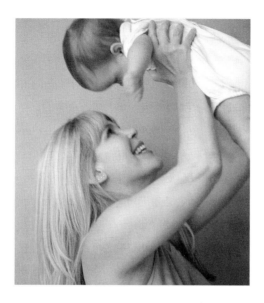

Kasey and Charly

Mom: Kasey, a first-time mom in her late thirties, is a former model. She had to overcome a long ordeal battling fertility obstacles before finally getting pregnant through in vitro fertilization. Because of the fertility hormones she'd received, she began her pregnancy several pounds over her normal weight. She had an uncomplicated pregnancy and was able to maintain a kickboxing and Pilates regimen throughout all three trimesters.

Charly: The photos were shot over several sessions between six and eight and a half months.

Delivery: C-section.

Started PeeWee Pilates: Eight weeks to the day after giving birth.

Kasey's impression of PeeWee Pilates: "I did everything I could to stay in shape throughout my pregnancy. Nonetheless, it was hell getting back into exercising. I had to take a lot of steps backward before I could get back to doing what I used to do almost effortlessly. Because of the extra pounds that I'm not used to carrying, I just didn't feel like myself. Nonetheless, I have to say that doing PeeWee Pilates with Charly has been so much fun in spite of the hard work for me. Charly views each session as her playtime, and her giggles keep me entertained."

Working with Kasey and Charly: Charly proved to be a dynamic and charismatic model, following in her model mother's footsteps. By the time we took these photos, she was an old PeeWee Pilates pro. She cheerfully arrived at the studio, greeted Holly with a big laugh, and crawled right to her pink mat, ready for action. Charly certainly brought home the point that eight-month-old babies are perfectly capable of learning a routine sequence and developing a clear sense of expectation about what is next to come. She exuberantly welcomed each exercise, sometimes joining in for the ride, sometimes trying to imitate her mom's movements, sometimes trying to anticipate which exercise came next. Sometimes, she'd become more infatuated with a nearby object and crawl over to grab it. Kasey would watch her carefully while moving through her exercises and would occasionally call her or stop to scoop her up if she veered too far away. At the end of each workout, as Kasey would quietly cool down and take a few moments in repose, Charly always mirrored her mom's shift in energy and tempo; she would snuggle up on top of or alongside Kasey and relax, too.

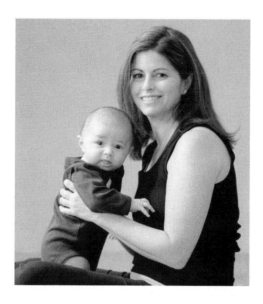

Cathy and Kyle

Mom: Cathy, a woman in her mid-thirties, left a career in the fashion industry to take care of her very active two-year-old son, Noah. During her pregnancy with her second child, she developed placenta previa and had to modify her activity level and increase bed rest for several months.

Kyle: Three and a half months at the time of the photo shoot.

Delivery: C-section.

Started PeeWee Pilates: At three months.

Cathy's impression of PeeWee Pilates: "The thing I love the most about these workouts is the time I get all alone with Kyle. It is so hard to find time in the day to just focus on him. I'm always so busy running after his brother. That makes these sessions feel special. The fact that I actually get to work on my own body is just an added benefit."

Working with Cathy and Kyle: We were very mindful of Cathy's recovery from her C-section, especially because she was still feeling somewhat sore and extremely fatigued. It took her some time to rebuild her stamina, most likely weakened by her prolonged ban on exercise during her pregnancy and her exhaustion taking care of an active toddler. She chose to start Pee-Wee Pilates slowly, following the C-section modifications. An experienced and relaxed mom, Cathy seemed especially comfortable moving about while holding Kyle. She made the task of balancing her attention to her own body with her focus on Kyle look effortless. Her easygoing, unflappable style matched Kyle's happy-go-lucky, calm demeanor. Like many three- or four-month-olds, Kyle was able to remain active and alert for long stretches of time while Kathy worked out, without fussing at all. At times, he was mesmerized by his face-to-face nonverbal exchanges with his mama; he would flash her his newfound social smile, gaze with great interest, and imitate her when she'd playfully stick out her tongue at him.